11-12-98

To Jane Louise,

Don't let the yeasties get you !

Carol

Who Killed Candida?

by
Vicki Glassburn

TEACH Services, Inc.
Brushton, New York 12916

© Copyright 1991 Vicki Glassburn
ISBN 0-945383-12-6 Paperback
ISBN 0-945383-28-2 Hard Cover
Library of Congress Catalog Number 89-51934

All rights reserved. First edition

Artwork by Neil Baker

If you would like information regarding reference books, suppliers of natural food, equipment, etc., please send a long, S.A.S.E. to:

VICTORY LIFESTYLES
P.O. Box 667
Marysville, Ohio 43040
(513) 644-0488

TEACH Services, Inc.
Donivan Road
RR 1 Box 182
Brushton, New York 12916

Dedication

Many people say that friends made during a war are the closest and that no one else can understand the strength of their bond. I can honestly say that I viewed my illness as a war between my mind and my body. Even though my mind rebelled against the confines of this disease, my body could not respond to my desire to be well.

I, too, made a friend during this war, one who shared my battle. Without her generosity and support, I truly doubt that I would be here today. She taught me, above all, to share this knowledge. Nancy, it is with much love that I dedicate this book to you.

Acknowledgements

I would like to thank:

My husband, for believing me when no one else did. Thank you for being my friend.

My mother, who is the most loyal, loving person I know. You were the only one who truly understood what I was going through.

My son, Tony, for his love, support, and humor. You were my inspiration to get well.

Charlie, who was the connecting factor in all of this. Your capacity to continually care about and help people is admirable. Thank you for your support.

Drs. Calvin and Agatha Thrash, of Uchee Pines Institute in Seale, Alabama, whose extensive research, study, and pursuance of natural therapies has provided a foundation for many of the principles in this book. God bless you for your work.

All of the Candida patients with whom I have shared this program. There is much joy in witnessing sick bodies regain health and, as a result, seeing all of you renew your love and zest for life. Put the anger and frustration associated with your illness behind you. Remember only enough to realize how precious our bodies are; treat them with kindness always.

Dr. Joseph D. Weissman, Assistant Professor of Medicine at UCLA and Author of *Choose To Live*, who maintains an active practice in Torrence, California.

Dr. William Crook, author of *The Yeast Connection*, for his support, input and continued interest in the Choices Conquer Candida (3-C) Program. Dr. Crook maintains an active practice in Jackson, Tennessee.

Most of all, I thank God for healing me.

Introduction

I would like to share with you a fantastic discovery: how to recover from Candida. What you will learn is that my battle with Candida was both the worst and the best experience I have ever gone through. After the pain and suffering came the healing; then came the opportunity to share how to conquer Candida by making better choices.

The Choices Conquer Candida (3-C)Program is unique in that it not only acknowledges a weakened immune system as part of a Candida problem but addresses the fact that an improperly functioning digestive system is also a factor. And, since a poor digestive system's ability to obtain maximum nutrients from food or supplements is greatly reduced, there exists little with which to nourish and support the immune system. Therefore, unless the digestive system is better regulated, recovery is often difficult to obtain. The 3-C Program comprehensively involves principles that restore the digestive system and rebuild the immune system. These same principles have been successfully used for many types of lifestyle-illnesses other than Candida.

The 3-C Program is comprised of two segments: "Getting Well" and "Staying Well." The program is low-cost and anyone can follow it. It involves a unique vegetarian diet, an all-natural anti-fungal extract, and various health principles that begin healing the immune system *immediately*, thereby reducing yeast colonization *immediately*!

The 3-C Program puts all of the pieces of the puzzle together. In the following pages you will share my experience with this devastating illness along with a few others who have successfully followed this program. Read on and discover how this program will allow you to do more than just "cope" with Candida, because — ***Choices Conquer Candida!***

Foreward

When I first met Vicki Glassburn, it was hard to believe that someone so full of life, so energetic, so obviously healthy, could have been the nightmarish person described in this book. The chronic Candidiasis syndrome is perhaps the prototypical lifestyle disease; in some people it causes only mild annoyances; in others it can be life-threatening, as in Vicki's case. The shattered immune system, apparently affected by toxins as well as many different allergens in the candida organism, allows dozens, if not hundreds, of environmental influences to batter the body. Few, if any, organ systems are spared. One can understand why many physicians would be extremely dubious that such wide-spread catastrophes could be possibly explained by one little organism — one which has heretofore been considered to be only a nuisance in a few people.

We all owe a tremendous debt of gratitude to Dr. Orian Truss, of Birmingham, Alabama, for formulating the theory of the chronic candida syndrome. And especially for carefully observing patients over a period of years — finding a consistent pattern, with consistent responses — before publishing his results. The Twentieth Century lifestyle factors of a chronically poor diet, heavy on sugars and other refined carbohydrates; the excessive use of potent antibiotics; the use of corticosteroids, often for minor problems; the near-universal use of "the pill" and other hormones; the widespread use of radiation and potent cancer chemotherapy are some of the factors that have caused this Twentieth Century scourge. Doubtless, if the candida organism had not attacked us, some other opportunistic organism would have.

What makes Vicki Glassburn's story so interesting is the fact that she had "tried everything" and failed. That in itself is not so surprising, since all of us who have had experience with this syndrome have seen patients who just did not respond. But Vicki did respond finally, and to a program that was very simple. Basically, it involved repairing the broken-down body defenses through very simple, natural methods — methods so simple that most people would feel that they were useless.

She was able to reverse the lifestyle insults very quickly when it seemed that nothing could help.

I am certain, and Vicki is absolutely convinced, that if she had not made sweeping changes in her diet and other lifestyle factors, she would not have recovered. And that is the reason Vicki has a real story to tell. I know that the reader will enjoy Vicki's story, and I believe that everyone will be greatly profited by her experience.

Calvin L. Thrash, M.D.

Preface

When this project first began, it contained much more technical information. However, in listening to many Candida patients (and as a former Candida patient), I came to realize how difficult it can be to concentrate when you don't feel well. In response to their suggestions, this book has been restructured into more of a "training manual." I hope that I have met our goal of outlining the program, including just enough information to somewhat substantiate the supporting theories so that you can first work toward your goal of getting well.

However, I hope your learning process will not stop there. Because I realize no one feels good about making changes in her (or his) lifestyle unless she (or he) is convinced the changes are worthwhile, I encourage you to pursue further study. The reference section of this book contains some resources that will provide more in-depth information concerning the principles of the 3-C Program, Candida, and illness in general.

I also hope that by the time you are through reading this book, the question "Who Killed Candida?" will be obvious. Killing Candida is not the issue; recovering health is.

Vicki

Table of Contents

CHAPTER 1

VICKI'S STORY

"What in the world did I do to deserve this?" I remember asking myself this question over and over during the course of a bizarre illness that, I realize now, came about little by little, over the years. I suppose the first culprit was the use of birth control pills on and off for ten years. Upon discontinuing them, I developed a poor complexion. My gynecologist commented that often after a woman discontinues birth control pills her normal hormone balance is not re-established. He recommended an endocrinologist, who used various hormones as a testing procedure and determined that, indeed, I had a hormone imbalance. Unfortunately, all he could offer was more hormone therapy. Out of frustration, I consulted a dermatologist who gave me a prescription for *Tetracycline*, stating that this antibiotic was safer than hormones. However, after six to eight months, *Tetracycline* seemed to lose its effectiveness.

Three years later, severe pre-menstrual syndrome (PMS) symptoms led to exploratory surgery that revealed a tumor and en-dometriosis. Treatment for these conditions included hormones, pain relievers, and anti-inflammatory medications. My condition worsened with repeated bladder infections and bowel problems. Consequently, six months later I underwent a total hysterectomy with bladder repair, including more anesthetics, pain relievers, and antibiotics. I was also started on estrogen therapy.

I was hospitalized again two weeks later because of a wide-spread infection that included the bladder. I had been on two different antibiotics for several days, but the doctor felt I now needed antibiotics intravenously. I developed symptoms that were attributed to an allergic reaction. Another antibiotic was administered, then another. Each one produced similar results. Finally, the infection was contained and I returned home. However, I soon discovered that any medication, even an aspirin, would produce adverse reactions. Only 20 to 30 minutes after taking the medicine I would develop flu-like symptoms, including headaches, joint pain, and depression. Then, after the symptoms subsided, I would fall into an almost coma-like sleep that would last for several hours.

At this point I knew something wasn't right. Why wasn't I getting better? I had been healthy all my life, always quick to recover from "common" surgeries such as appendectomy, tonsillectomy, sinus surgery, and tubal ligation. My only nagging complaints were sinus headaches and hypoglycemia symptoms, such as occasional fatigue. I thought my diet was healthier than that of most people, I was exercising regularly, and I had even stopped smoking.

New symptoms began to develop. A dull, pulsating sound in my head appeared over the next several weeks. It was as if I could hear my heart beating in my skull. Have you ever laid your head on your pillow in a certain position and heard that sound? My hearing became very sensitive, and loud noises began to bother me. I also noticed a numb sensation in my left hand every time I raised my arm.

I returned to work after a seven-week surgery leave. Even though I felt better than before the surgery, I still wasn't myself. I thought all I needed was a little more time to get back to normal. Over the next several weeks, the pulsating sensation in my head worsened, and I had to turn the television volume up just to drown it out. Sporadic headaches would appear, plus attacks of sudden dizziness. Some time later, I also noticed that I had visual disturbances, "seeing" something in my peripheral vision that really wasn't there. These "dark patches" came and went in addition to white spots (sometimes referred to as "floaters") that were constantly in front of my eyes.

My gynecologist assured me these symptoms were not a result of my hysterectomy; however, he did increase my estrogen dosage several times until I reached the highest recommended limit. He recommended I consult a specialist.

A neurologist listened to my symptoms and seemed very concerned. He thought I could have any one of several serious problems, including a brain tumor or an artery malfunction, such as an aneurysm. He said I needed an angiogram, in which a substance called "dye" would be injected into my veins in order to locate the arterial malfunction. Realizing that these invasive tests always carry a risk, in addition to the fact that I had experienced an adverse reaction to a dye injection years before, I told him I would rather wait a few weeks to see if these symptoms would possibly clear up on their own. He insisted that another test, a brain CAT Scan (Computerized Axial Tomography), be performed. He said this test would not require the use of dye but rather a "contrast medium" injected into my veins to scan the arteries of the brain. He said this procedure would not carry the risk of an angiogram.

Even though I was leery of the possible dangers of these tests, the prospect of an aneurysm was equally as foreboding and the experiences of several of my acquaintances came to mind. Years earlier my cousin had died of an aneurysm, and more recently, two women in my golf league had experienced aneurysms – and only one survived.

About this time I experienced yet another symptom: a grinding noise each time I moved my eyes from side to side. My headaches worsened and I became more and more frightened. Fearing that the doctor was right concerning the possibility of an aneurysm, I decided I had better find out exactly what I was dealing with. So approximately one week later, a CAT Scan was performed. As the attendant began injecting the second bottle of contrast medium, I began to feel really strange. My whole body felt like it was starting to swell. Then I noticed a strange sensation in my throat, as though it also was swelling, closing off my air supply. I mentioned to the attendant that I was having trouble breathing and he immediately disconnected the contrast medium supply and called for a doctor. My chest felt as though it had a tight metal band around it, and I couldn't take a deep breath. Soon I couldn't breathe at all. I remember seeing the look of panic on the technician's face and thinking to myself, "So this is what it feels like to die."

After losing consciousness, I awoke to an equally frightening experience. My heart felt as though it was going to explode out of my chest as several doctors administered first Adrenalin, then Benadryl. Combined, these two substances produced a strong burning sensation in my throat; however, they did counteract the allergic reaction.

Once stabilized, I was quickly pushed into the X-ray chamber. The doctors were hopeful that there was enough of the contrast medium left in my brain to verify an arterial malfunction. Realizing that future injections of this substance could possibly be fatal, they felt it would be the last chance to find the possible aneurysm. During this procedure, I couldn't figure out why the technician kept referring to the contrast medium as "dye." I explained to him that my neurologist specifically said I would be given a contrast medium, which was different than dye. Much to my dismay, the technician informed me that they were one and the same and that I should never submit to either one again.

I could not return home because I continued to experience symptoms similar to those I had during the initial allergic reaction. Every hour or so, my chest would become very tight and I felt as though my throat was swelling shut, cutting off my air supply. This experience was also accompanied by a metallic taste in my mouth. These "attacks" lasted from 10 to 15 minutes and scared me beyond belief. Every time I experienced one, I was afraid my heart would stop. The attacks continued, on and off, for 24 hours, decreasing in severity. Finally, by the next morning they were gone, or so I thought.

Returning to work the next day, I noticed that going into the printing department of my place of employment brought back this constricting feeling in my throat, a heaviness in my chest, and an inability to breathe. I couldn't believe this was happening to me! I tried to convince myself that it would just take a few days to recover from the allergic reaction; however, my sensitivities grew worse instead of better. Everywhere I went there seemed to be substances that evoked these reactions: the chemicals in the printing department and research lab, the cleaning fluids used by the maintenance crew, chemicals used in lawn care outside, materials used in newly remodeled departments, and even the smoke, perfume, and cologne of my co-workers produced this reaction. I tried to explain this to fellow employees, but no one seemed to understand what I was talking about. They would only say, "What do you mean, your throat is swelling shut and you can't breathe?"

Later that day I contacted the neurologist to find out if the X-rays were conclusive. Unfortunately, he said they were not, and since my symptoms had remained, he insisted on performing an angiogram. I couldn't believe he would even suggest this! When I reminded him of my near-fatal reaction to the dye, he casually said, "No problem; we'll just load you up with so much cortisone to suppress the immune system, you won't react to anything."

He also mentioned that because of increasing symptoms of poor coordination, numbness, and tingling sensations in my extremities, he suspected the beginning of an autoimmune disease—muscular dystrophy. I asked him if the pounding in my head could possibly have something to do with my ear, especially since my hearing had become super sensitive. It seemed as though I had a microphone in my ear that intensified all noises, including the pounding in my head, which I could now hear above a room full of people. Concentrating at work became difficult, and sleeping was almost impossible. I was constantly tired and had never experienced fear like this before. It seemed to consume my whole life. I convinced the neurologist to let me consult with an eye, ear, nose and throat specialist. Then, if the symptoms were not gone within three weeks, I would agree to the angiogram.

I really never had any intention of permitting him to perform the angiogram because I knew I would never survive another injection of dye. I decided I would rather take my chances with an aneurysm than die from a fatal allergic reaction.

The eye, ear, nose, and throat specialist was not optimistic, to say the least. He explained that the sound I was hearing probably was my heart beating and that it very likely was due to an aneurysm involving a main artery behind my middle ear. He, like the neurologist, suggested I have an angiogram as soon as possible: another dead end.

In the meantime, I had been hearing a lot about a dental-related condition known as TMJ (Temporal Mandibular Joint), which is a misalignment of the jaw that can produce headaches, ringing in the ears, and many other problems of the face and head. Since years earlier I had been diagnosed with a severe overbite, I prayed that something this simple would prove to be my problem. Instead of going back to the neurologist, I contacted a TMJ specialist. After a thorough examination and extensive X-rays, she concluded that I did, indeed, have a misalignment of the jaw. This specialist felt confident that my headaches and the pounding sensations would recede as our treatment progressed. I was overjoyed! She outlined a two-year plan that would include wearing a plastic "splint" in my mouth, which would gradually force my jaw back into its proper position. I was supposed to return at two-week intervals to have the splint readjusted as my jaw muscles adapted. Then, after approximately one year, she planned to fit me with braces to better adjust my teeth to match the new position of my jaw. There was only one problem with this treatment program: repositioning the splint required pouring a chemical liquid, acrylic, onto the splint, then holding it in my mouth until it dried. During the very first treatment, I had a severe allergic reaction and could not continue the program — more wasted time and money, to say nothing of the the emotional letdown.

Shortly thereafter, my mother told me about a television program she had seen concerning people who suffered from a syndrome similar to mine. They, too, experienced strange symptoms that didn't seem to relate to any specific illness. She sent for a book about this condition and passed it on to me. It was called *The Yeast Connection* by Dr. William Crook. I read that many people with symptoms like mine suffer from an overabundance of a particular strain of yeast known as *Candida albicans*. This condition is commonly referred to as Candida. I was encouraged to find that I was not alone in my sickness and heartened to know that a program offering relief was available!

I immediately put myself on Dr. Crook's recommended program, including the Candida Control Diet and supplements outlined in his book. I also contacted his office for the name of a clinical ecologist/allergist specializing in Candida treatment in my area. With only three such doctors in the entire state, I felt fortunate that one was located 45 minutes away. But, due to his very busy schedule, I had to wait over a month for an appointment. In the meantime, I did not notice any improvement in my symptoms utilizing the Candida Control Diet and other suggestions in Dr. Crook's book. Therefore, I switched to the more severe diet he recommended called the Low Carbohydrate Diet. (Dr. Crook has since made revisions in subsequent reprintings of this book. The diets I followed were from the first edition.)

On the day of my appointment with the Candida specialist, I was fully examined and thoroughly questioned concerning my health history and symptoms. By then I could add to my list of symptoms a vaginal discharge and worsening of a long-standing sinus condition for which I had already undergone one surgery. Although the specialist indicated I possibly had a yeast overgrowth problem, he wasn't sure by examination alone. Comprehensive allergy testing revealed that I was allergic to several different foods, including yeast, and many inhalants. Therefore, a blood sample was sent to a laboratory to obtain a more specific yeast level evaluation. Realizing it would take approximately one month for the yeast test results, I continued with the prescribed diet and other recommendations.

Little by little, I began to notice that I was becoming allergic to additional foods, perfumes, and freshly cut grass. Coming into contact with these elements produced a "heavy chest" feeling and a tightening of the throat that made it difficult to breathe. I could also detect mold and mildew in places such as bathrooms, basements, and even outdoors that other people could not smell.

The doctor and I were both surprised that the results of the yeast test showed that I not only had Candida, but a very considerable amount of it. In fact, my yeast count was over 400 while a normal count is approximately 80. He prescribed nystatin, which is a widely-used antifungal medication, and started testing procedures to develop a yeast vaccine appropriate for my immune system. In addition to being on Dr. Crook's Low Carbohydrate Diet, I had taken it upon myself to totally give up all fruit and high-carbohydrate vegetables. My Candida specialist further restricted my diet by eliminating grains. However, with each passing week I found myself tolerating even fewer foods and chemicals as this illness chipped away at my immune system.

Sometimes the chips were more like big chunks. For example, new carpet was being installed down the hall from my office area at work, and the odor of the carpet made me nauseous all morning.

However, when the carpet adhesive was spread on the floor, my throat started to close up, my chest began to hurt, and I felt like I couldn't breathe. My doctor later confirmed that this was an "asthma" attack. After I left the building for about 30 minutes, my symptoms subsided; however, they started again each time I tried to re-enter the building. I called the Candida specialist and he explained that each time large amounts of chemicals entered my system, the reactions worsened. Because of my weakened immune system, he advised me not to return to work until the chemical fumes had dissipated. I knew that would take some time, especially since the building did not have windows that could be opened.

The situation at home was better than at work for a while, but then it, too, became a nightmare. In order to cope with my chemical allergies, I had to make the following changes:

—I could not drive my new car due to my allergies to the chemicals in many of the interior products. (However, if an item had "outgassed", meaning it had already discharged a great deal of its molecules, it would be more tolerable). For this reason, driving an older car was more tolerable for me. Even in an older car, I was limited to low-traffic areas due to the exhaust fumes from other cars.

—I purchased special carbon filter masks to use against exposure to chemicals, exhaust fumes, plastics, mold in flower beds, and new merchandise in stores. I quickly learned to go nowhere without one.

—Inks and carbons of all types became offensive, including newsprint, ballpoint pens, carbon paper, photocopies, and felt-tip markers. Close contact with these items would make me sick for several hours; therefore, I tried to avoid them as much as possible. I could only use my typewriter near an open window because of the electrical fumes.

—I removed from my home every plastic and vinyl product that I possibly could. I replaced all Tupperware-type containers with glass containers. Several months earlier, we had added an extra bath to our home, which contained many vinyl products: flooring, wall coverings, shower unit, and sink top. Due to the outgassing of these and the new wood, I had to keep the door closed and sealed with towels in order to use my kitchen, even though these two rooms were separated by a utility room! Two-year-old vinyl shades in my bedroom were tolerable only if I left them rolled up.

—Other synthetic materials in the form of woven goods were also a problem. It was necessary for me to replace acrylic-backed or synthetic-blend drapes, synthetic-blend clothing, latex-backed rugs, mattresses, sheets, blankets, pillows, and bedspreads. The only way I could tolerate washing new or synthetic items for my family was by wearing my mask as I threw them into the washer and hung them outside to dry.

—I disposed of all household cleansers, candles, waxes, laundry detergents, cosmetics, and items such as deodorant soaps and perfumed shampoos. I put my perfumes in sealed containers, hoping someday to be able to use them again. My husband removed all paint, varnish, insecticides, fertilizers, weed killers, and other various chemicals from our garage, because I could actually detect them through the walls of our house. I searched, usually unsuccessfully, for alternative brands of cleansers, toiletry items, and cosmetics that contained no offensive odor.

—In an effort to reduce my exposure to mold, my doctor recommended that I remove all plants from the house. After giving away all of my plants, I discovered that "spider plants" were beneficial in eliminating the formaldehyde from outgassed vinyl and plastic products. Since formaldehyde was a major chemical allergen for me, I purchased several of these beneficial plants and added a newly-discovered mold-inhibitor to the soil. Also, due to mold, I could not tolerate burning wood, leaves, or freshly-cut grass. It was sheer terror every time I heard one of our neighbors start a lawn mower. I would immediately make arrangements to leave the neighborhood. Usually, my mother would pick me up because I could tolerate her car. Then, I always had to stay out of the neighborhood for several hours until the pollen settled.

—Fumes from fireplaces, coal burners, and even gas furnaces bothered me. I was thankful that it became summer as my condition worsened, eliminating the need for a heating system. However, as the weather warmed, I found I could not even tolerate our air conditioning due to the mold that typically accumulates in these units.

—Tobacco smoke of all kinds was probably my worst enemy. Whether I was exposed to it directly or indirectly (on someone's clothing), these substances produced violent reactions. When my husband came home from work, he would immediately have to change his clothes due to cigarette smoke and/or chemicals used at his place of employment. Smoke was tolerable only at social functions that were held outside.

I tried to keep all of these substances out of my environment as best I could. However, my only really "safe" haven was at the office of the Candida specialist, where I never had to worry about exposure to chemicals. I remember actually looking forward to upcoming appointments, because no one there wore perfume or smoked, there were no chemically-scented air fresheners, new furniture, or fabrics to outgas. The doctor and his wonderful staff were understanding and did all they could to help Candida patients like me. I tried to sound very positive and optimistic when I spoke to them so that my treatment program would move along as quickly as possible. I was especially anxious to start yeast vaccine therapy because it had been successful for a few other patients. With each subsequent visit I hoped there would be some new discovery that would hasten my recovery. Unfortunately, this was not the case, and I continued to worsen.

Even more depressing were the other environmentally-ill people at this clinic who had been suffering much longer than I. Some of them were forced to give up their livelihood and, like me, become a recluse at home. One lady spoke of stripping her newly-built home down to the wooden studs so it could be lined with a special foil covering to prevent chemical outgassing. A college professor could only teach on a substitute basis if she first went to the school and made sure there were no offensive chemical odors. She had worked very hard to get her PhD, and now she was forced to teach at an elementary level. She said elementary teaching posed fewer problems because the younger children didn't ask so many questions, especially if she had to wear a filter face mask. She cried as she told me how many times she had to suddenly leave a school because of exposures to cleaning chemicals used by either the janitor or kitchen staff.

Some of these poor people were struggling through their food allergies only by using "food drops," which enabled them to eat the foods they were allergic to every four to ten days. Otherwise, they would have a terrible reaction and not be able to tolerate these foods at all. I, also, obtained food drops through another doctor. These drops helped my immune system tolerate a certain food in the same manner.

Personnel at the company where I was employed had never heard of Candida and had difficulty believing I was truly ill. Keep in mind that I experienced this illness several years ago. At that time, only two books, *The Yeast Connection* and *The Missing Link*, plus a few obscure magazine or medical journal articles on Candida were available to the public. My employer contacted my doctor several times to question and re-question him about the validity of my condition. My doctor answered all their questions and did his best to explain my illness. We made available to them all information that we had on Candida. However, my employer still wanted to classify my leave as "personal" rather than medical. My co-workers also did not understand this illness. Many of them thought I was merely suffering from the after-effects of a hysterectomy or that I simply wanted some time off from work with pay.

They did not understand how much I wanted to be "normal" again. If I were going to fake an illness, why would I pick such an unusual, bizarre one? If all I wanted was time off with pay, I could have returned to the neurologist and officially obtained the diagnosis of muuscular dystrophy, especially since my coordination problems and muscular weaknesses were worsening. (These are very often common symptoms of yeast-related illness.) I wanted to return to work so much that I even asked my employer to allow me to use a portable oxygen tank at work because other chemically-sensitive patients told me that's how they survived certain environments. My doctor agreed that oxygen would alleviate breathing problems; however, the company would not permit its use due to their safety regulations. I found it difficult trying to verify my illness and explain various treatment methods to my employer. I tried to remain optimistic in spite of the depression I felt.

I continued to increase my nystatin dosage as fast as the Candida specialist would permit. I was willing to make myself even more sick due to "die off" if it would kill the yeast faster. (Die-off is a term used to signify that yeast is being reduced, which will be covered in Chapter 2.) I never, never cheated on the diet, no matter how sick I was of eating the same meats and vegetables. A side effect of the nystatin was nausea, which also made mealtimes unappealing. I never had a single dessert, piece of fruit, yeast product, cheese — nothing that wasn't allowed. Whatever the doctor said to do, I did one better. I even convinced him to give me yeast extract shots sooner than he normally would have. This therapy is designed to stimulate the body to fight off the yeast on its own. However, the difficulty was in finding just the right dosage. My reactions to this vaccine included nausea, weakness, and disorientation. But I was willing to do anything just to get well.

The nystatin medication was not producing the "miracle" results I had read about. I did notice a relief from sporadic headaches and a slight decrease in the numbness and tingling in my arms and legs, but those improvements only seemed a trade-off for increased allergic reactions to so many things that I sometimes couldn't tell what was making me sick. Was it one of the recommended medicines or supplements such as nystatin, estrogen, vitamins, minerals, acidophilus, garlic oil capsules, linseed oil, or was it a food or chemical?

Even the yeast in factory-canned products can make a Candida patient very ill, so I purchased organic vegetables. In order to eliminate mold or mildew, vegetables that were not organic had to first be washed in a diluted Clorox bath, then rinsed several times. This was difficult to tolerate, even with a mask on.

Due to the fact that my employer insisted my illness was "personal," I had gone without several paychecks, and my financial situation became a hardship that affected the entire family. Eventually, my employer did consider my illness a medical condition and I was compensated. I was also grateful that my husband and I both had medical insurance through our employers. However, we were still responsible for all deductibles as well as portions of every doctor visit, test, or medication. Because a great deal of the expenses encountered by Candida sufferers are not covered by insurance, the financial burden can be overwhelming. This is especially true for those who are chemically sensitive. Some of the expenses involved are:

—Replacing items made with synthetic fabrics with natural materials. Some of these items included clothing, linens, blankets, pillows, bedspreads, rugs, and curtains. Some patients even have to replace larger items such as mattresses, wallpaper, furniture, and carpeting. Even though our carpeting was two years old, the odor from the stain protector finish had to be removed via a steam cleaning process in order for me to stay in my home.

—Replacing a large portion of vinyl or plastic items, such as drinking glasses, dishes, storage containers, trash cans, furniture, vinyl-coated wallpaper, window shades, mini-blinds — the list goes on and on. So many items in an average home contain vinyl or plastic! If an item was old and had outgassed, I could sometimes tolerate it. However, some items that were old still bothered me, while some were tolerable as long as they weren't close to me. (I remember having a huge yard sale and trying to explain to everyone why I was selling so many items from my home that were new or nearly new!)

—Replacing soap, laundry detergents, household cleansers, and other such items with products that contained no perfumes or chemicals was necessary, but difficult. These products are not readily available, and had to be ordered from specialty stores or catalogs. While companies that manufacture these products provide a valuable service to persons like me, their products are usually very expensive.

—Purchasing items that assist Candida patients in tolerating their environment, such as charcoal filter masks, air purifiers, and replacement filters. Many patients even find it necessary to either remove or cover the walls or floors in their home with a special foil material. Naturally, all of these items are especially expensive.

—Purchasing organically-grown foods was necessary to reduce further exposure to chemicals. In addition to being very expensive, they were often difficult to locate. For the same reason, I purchased or obtained only bottled distilled water.

—Purchasing numerous nutritional dietary supplements such as vitamins, minerals, herbs, and other items conducive to a Candida treatment program such as linseed oil, garlic oil capsules, nystatin and hydrogen peroxide.

—Other miscellaneous expenses included long-distance telephone calls to doctors' offices, nutritionists, health food stores, distributors, and other individuals knowledgeable in the area of Candida. Additionally, insurance did not cover alternative therapy expenses for massage, reflexology, and colonic treatments.

In addition to coping with adjustments in my home environment, I also had to deal with the obscurity of this illness. Unfortunately, only a few enlightened doctors knew much about this "new disease of the '80s," as it later became known. They could adequately describe to me what Candida is, and how my exposure to so many medications had led me to this point; however, they were not helpful in treating it. Even though I did find information on what Candida was, the problem was how to control it. For some, the "typical" treatment programs were helpful, but for many others, including me, they were not. There were no support groups in my town, so I struck out on my own to call or write other support groups or anyone who had knowledge of alternative therapies. I purchased what few books were available and ordered reprints of every article I either read or heard about that offered additional information. I attended a natural healing center where massage, reflexology, colonics, and vitamin/herb therapy were applied.

The author of a Candida cookbook suggested I add large quantities of linseed oil and butter to my diet to keep from losing more weight. Although I had always been petite (my normal weight was slightly over 100 pounds), I lost even more weight due to a limited diet. It seemed that nearly every food was forbidden because of allergies and the Low Carbohydrate Diet. I used a small bottle of linseed oil every two days and consumed one-half stick of butter with every meal. I was desperate to keep my weight up since my doctor had said if I continued to lose weight he would add more high-carbohydrate, high-calorie foods back into my diet. At that time, it was a widely accepted fact that those foods were the ones that supposedly "fed the yeast"; therefore, if I ate them, my Candida symptoms, especially the chemical sensitivities, would worsen. In addition, I increased my garlic oil capsule dosage from eight to twelve per day as I continued to read of its wonderful antifungal properties.

My depression increased and my memory worsened day by day. It was hard to remain optimistic and happy when it was so difficult to complete even the simplest tasks. As an example, my husband called from work one morning and asked if I could put leftovers in the oven for his lunch. As I turned my attention to something else, I promptly forgot his call and went back to bed. I no longer had the energy for housework and found that my daily chores were almost more than I could handle. In an effort to keep my environment chemical-free, I had to locate, purchase, and store organic foods and cook for myself. I would drag myself to the microwave, then to the table to eat, take my supplements and medicine, and then go back to bed.

Between my physical condition, our financial situation, and the hopelessness of it all, life was pretty depressing. I became a recluse because I could hardly tolerate the chemicals that were everywhere in my environment. On many occasions I tried to go out with my family, but there was always some substance that would cause me to leave. Either smoke, perfume, deodorant, cologne, car fumes, lawns being mowed or fertilized, or God-knows-what would send me packing. What most people didn't realize is that certain conditions could fluctuate. For example, I could enter a store one day and be fine. However, the next day that same store could stock new merchandise that emitted certain chemicals to which I was allergic. This was especially true for clothing and all types of vinyl and plastic. I could tolerate a grocery store pretty well, except for the aisle that contained household cleaners and laundry detergents. I could spend time at a golf course only if no chemical lawn care treatment had been applied within the last few days. My reactions to any of these substances included a tightening of my chest and throat to the point that I thought I could no longer breathe and I would become asthmatic. I also became dizzy, disoriented, and nauseous. I became so weak that I could barely lift the groceries out of the cart. When I returned home, that "little trip" would have me in bed for hours. I finally reached the point where I had to stay out of most stores altogether.

My husband and son watched me deteriorate, mentally as well as physically. Other members of my family did not understand what I was going through, with the exception of my mother, so it was hard for them to know what to do or say. My friends also stayed away for this reason. Hardly anyone called or came to see me. The few people I did see did not understand about Candida or chemical and environmental allergies. All they knew was that I looked like "death warmed over." Much of my hair had turned gray during this illness, and my weight was now down to approximately 79 pounds.

Unfortunately, as I became more sensitive, I found that I could no longer tolerate even the small amount of chemicals that remained in my home. Exposure to items that I could previously handle, such as odors from the couch, the garage, and vinyl wallpaper, became unbearable. Because my illness had already disrupted my family's life so much, I did not want them to make further changes by totally stripping what was left of our home. In addition, other chemically sensitive patients had informed me that it is nearly impossible to remove every single exposure to chemicals.

Due to these factors, I looked into the possibility of moving into a sterile environment facility for chemically allergic patients. In effect, I would be living in a "bubble" that would protect what was left of my immune system from dangerous exposures. It was very expensive and I cried at the thought of leaving my family and living life as even more of a recluse than I had been. Even though I normally was a very optimistic person, the frustration and hopelessness of this illness seemed to change my entire outlook on life. Caught between the fears of a fatal chemical exposure and the fact that I might actually have an aneurysm (the pounding in my head was relentless), I actually contemplated suicide. My distorted reasoning was, "I'm going to die anyway; why not hurry death along so my family won't have to put up with me any longer!"

One day, as I was struggling to cook my lunch, I received a phone call from a friend of mine. Despite my frustration with this illness, I always tried to remain cheerful on the phone because I knew that some people thought my problems were merely emotional, a result of having a hysterectomy. I thought that if I sounded positive, people would be more inclined to believe my illness was real. My friend wanted to let me know that she had asked her Sunday School class to pray for my recovery. Although I appreciated her concern, I hadn't attended church for several years and, in the face of this illness, felt as though God had deserted me. Yet, I was so touched by her compassion that I sat down and cried. Lately it seemed that all I did was cry.

A few minutes later, I received another phone call that changed my life. I heard about a lady who had been ill several years earlier with similar symptoms. A doctor had given her a diet known as the "Pancreas Recovery Diet," which she used to regain her health. I contacted her and listened as she described not only her recovery but also how she had gathered information from several conditioning centers that taught lifestyle changes. She had incorporated these two programs and research of her own into a new recovery program. She graciously invited me to her home to assist me in learning this recovery program. Even though I was skeptical of the simplicity of this program, I realized that I really had no other options available.

The environment in her home posed problems for me. Because of the presence of mold and mildew, I could not sleep in the bedroom in the basement. Even though this may not have been detected by most people, to me it was intolerable. I was so sensitive that I had allergic reactions to the "dust" from whole wheat flour being milled, chopped fresh onions, chlorine in the swimming pool, and on and on. I even reacted to being out in the sun at first. I turned red from head to toe and small, itchy bumps appeared all over my body.

The program that she began to teach me was so different from what I had been accustomed to I could hardly believe it would be successful; it seemed too simple, too natural. However, I was willing to try anything. Therefore, in spite of my extreme fatigue, I forced myself to follow the requirements: exercising every day whether I felt like it or not, spending time in the sun, drinking lots of a certain type of water, and utilizing a whole new diet. I also learned the importance of a properly functioning digestive system and all of the associated principles behind this theory.

Due to changing my diet and other components of the program, I experienced severe die-off initially. I was strongly encouraged to discontinue taking nystatin and the hormone estrogen. Even though nystatin is an antifungal antibiotic that will reduce yeast, I also knew that other antibiotics can actually contribute to yeast overgrowth and I simply felt an all-natural antifungal would accomplish the same thing without damaging my immune system. In fact, the all-natural antifungal recommended by this new program allowed my immune system to fight the Candida on its own.

Exercising took all the strength I could gather. I was so weak that, had I been at home, I am sure I would have said "forget it" and stayed on the couch. However, within a week, even though not physically well, I felt as though a "fog" had lifted from my mind. Within two weeks, my memory was definitely better. My energy returned slowly, day by day, apparent as my walking distances improved. I began to learn how the human body is supposed to function, compared to how it is often forced to function. Within a few weeks, I felt so much better that I wanted to return home, despite objections. I was so excited about my improvement to-date that I wanted to get home as soon as possible to show my family that I had begun to get better. Can you imagine feeling hope for the first time? I was eager to continue the program at home so that I could eventually go back to work and become "normal" again, being able to go anywhere I wanted and be able to associate with anyone I chose, without experiencing allergic reactions.

So home I went, promising to strictly adhere to this new lifestyle. I received the promise that doing so would ensure that the rest of my allergies would gradually disappear, and I would soon be well. And I was! Within one month, my chemical allergies were much improved and I could eat all sorts of foods I had previously been allergic to. In another month, I returned to work to find that my department was being renovated, including the staining and varnishing of new doors and installation of new vinyl-coated walls. Even though I had some slight symptoms of allergic reactions, I was able to tolerate them, and within another month, even those were gone!

Can you imagine how I felt as I regained not only my health, but my life? It was truly amazing that a program so simple and natural had achieved what 17 different doctors plus various products, treatments, and techniques could not. Naturally, I was totally committed to this program and never cheated. Not only had it alleviated my allergies and other ailments associated with Candida, but other pre-existing conditions such as sinusitis and an overbite. Since childhood, I had suffered with various sinus symptoms, including headaches, pain around my eyes, difficulty in breathing through my nose, and runny nose. I had even undergone a sinus surgery, which only improved my condition temporarily, and was contemplating another. However, all of these symptoms disappeared within two months of initiating this program. More surprising was the fact that this diet was instrumental in correcting the misalignment of my jaw that I had been aware of for at least 10 years. After a few months on this program, I noticed that my bite felt different and, upon consulting a dentist, he remarked that I no longer had an overbite. Eventually, we realized that something was forcing my jaw back into its proper position. That something, we decided, must be the nutritious diet I was on. After all, if a proper diet contributes to good muscle tone throughout the body, wouldn't this also include the muscles of the jaw? Another health benefit was healthier hair that looked better than it had in months.

Needless to say, I was very dedicated to this program and never felt better in my life. Not only did I lose all existing allergies, but I had immense energy. My previous days filled with fatigue, when I could do little more than lie on the couch, were exchanged for extremely active days that began at 5:00 AM and ended at 9:00 PM. I was able to return to work full time, as well as take care of my family and home, cook and go shopping, and became socially active again. Additionally, I took on a part-time job as well as spending many hours on the phone each week sharing this wonderful program with other Candida patients.

The Candida specialist was totally surprised when I reported my dramatic recovery to him. A follow-up blood test to measure yeast levels in my body confirmed that my yeast count was now back in the normal range; all this after only four months! I visited with him for two hours to share this program in hopes that he would be interested in including it in his treatment of others. Although interested, he was very skeptical and even charged for the visit!

I started sharing what I had learned with others and tried to help them understand that Candida is not their sole health problem. Candida does not cause a weakened immune system; rather, it is a result of a weakened immune system. Instead of focusing on "killing yeast," Candida patients first need to focus on rebuilding and strengthening their immune system. Once this is accomplished, a properly functioning immune system will not allow an overgrowth of any harmful microorganisms.

In the following pages, you will read the abbreviated stories of just a few of many other people who also found that changing their lifestyles renewed their health and vitality in addition to conquering Candida. Please keep in mind that while all of these stories are absolutely true, restoring one's health does not occur overnite. Each of these individuals, as well as I, achieved health success through a constant dedication to the 3-C Program.

Connie

At this moment it's hard for me to remember the last time I really didn't feel well, but several years ago, it was impossible for me to remember the last time I felt good. I've been on Vicki's 3-C Program for the past three years now, and I'm enjoying incredibly good health for the first time since I started college in 1977.

Most illnesses start out on a small scale, so much so that you don't notice all the signals that your body is sick. After graduating from high school, I went away to college where, in addition to all my classes, I had a full-time job and an apartment to keep up. I never took time to eat right and felt I couldn't afford nutritious foods. I hardly slept because in addition to my hectic work and school schedule I also partied a lot, staying up late and drinking alcohol and smoking. In addition, I was taking birth control pills and eating *Pepto Bismol* and *Rolaids* like they were candy. I suffered from diarrhea, gas, stomach cramps, and was severely anemic. This went on for two years; then I dropped out of school and moved to Florida, hoping a change of scenery would improve my life. However, I still drank a lot of alcohol, ate lots of sweet foods, and rarely exercised; soon I had gained 60 pounds and a peptic ulcer.

Finding no relief in Florida, I moved back to Ohio where, for the next eight years, my stomach problems became progressively worse. I consulted with at least ten different doctors in an attempt to determine exactly what was wrong with me. Each one handed me more prescriptions for various bowel relaxants, laxatives, sleeping pills, and antibiotics (for conditions such as colds, bronchitis, sinus infections, yeast infections, flu, and irritable bowel syndrome). I was also on birth control pills for ten years until my hair started to fall out. I went through every test imaginable, including upper and lower GI's, CAT scans, magnetic resonance tests, and X-rays. For ten years, the diarrhea and severe constipation would alternate. I developed fibroid cysts in both breasts and had to have several aspirations. I also kept postponing a recommended D & C (dilation and curettage). I was depressed, overweight, and agonized over increasing hair loss.

My social life became practically non-existent due to constant and severe gas, bloating, abdominal pain, and diarrhea. I spent all of my time either at work or at my parents' home. Beginning a new job at an automobile factory caused me to be constantly exposed to many petrochemicals, such as paint fumes, dyes, and forklift exhaust fumes, and much dirt and dust. Before long, I began to experience all kinds of weird symptoms such as asthma attacks, dizziness, forgetfulness, sudden and explosive mood swings, depression, skin rashes, and mild panic attacks.

Four years later, I developed cancer. Hearing this diagnosis from my doctor was the most terrifying thing I could ever imagine. I had melanoma carcinoma, which is a rare type of skin cancer that can infect the lymphatic system very quickly and can be very deadly. Here I was, only thirty years old with a very bleak outlook. I endured two surgeries and a dozen biopsies over the next six months. My doctor informed me that I would probably face a cancer surgery every year. His only recommendation was to try a vigorous chemotherapy treatment, which could possibly extend my life somewhat. I lost 20 pounds, my boyfriend, my sense of humor, and any hope for the future. Additionally, I began to develop acute allergic reactions to all sorts of things that never bothered me prior to my surgeries. The panic attacks became so severe that I actually missed six weeks of work because I was afraid to leave my house. A doctor at a local mental health facility gave me a prescription for *Xanax*, an anti-depressant. As the irritable bowel symptoms worsened, I lived on *7-Up* and saltine crackers for weeks because it was all I could keep down or digest. Not realizing the damage I was doing, I ate boxes of *Pepto-Bismol* tablets and drank bottles of *Kaopectate* to combat constant diarrhea.

Six months earlier, my mother had suggested that I call Vicki, but I kept putting it off. I had read Dr. Crook's book, *The Yeast Connection*, and visited an allergist who put me on *Capristatin*, an antifungal, which seemed to help for only a few weeks. He recommended eating a lot of meat, which did not seem to agree with me.

One day, after crying myself to sleep, I awoke so violently ill that I really wished I would just die and get it over with. I didn't know how much longer I could live like this. Desperate, I called Vicki. She was the warmest and most caring person I had talked to and seemed to truly understand my illness. As she explained her program to me, I realized that there was really nothing left for me. I was too afraid to try any more medication. Calling Vicki was the start of a new beginning for me and I truly feel her program saved my life. Her positive attitude and energy was an inspiration. I am also grateful for the support of my family.

However, I was probably one of Vicki's most stubborn clients initially. Not fully understanding that this was a truly comprehensive program, I sometimes did not follow the diet properly or make all of the necessary lifestyle changes. For instance, a couple of times I got really daring and resorted to my old eating habits, which would sometimes result in getting a cold or flu, stomach and bowel upsets, and another reprimand from Vicki! Why did I cheat? I think that being sick for such a long time, taking lots of medication and seeking help from so many sources makes one assume that simple changes such as diet, good water, exercise, and digestion principles could never truly conquer serious health problems. However, after several espisodes of cheating, I was becoming more and more convinced that whatever it was that "I felt like I had to eat" was not worth what I went through physically afterwards. I finally convinced myself over the months that feeling great was a worthy exchange for eating healthy foods.

Initially I did experience severe die-off using the *Kyolic* liquid garlic, but then I began to feel better. In fact, I noticed an improvement as soon as I gave up meat. It seemed that the more carefully I followed

Vicki's suggestions, the better I felt. Symptoms such as allergies, panic attacks, diarrhea (except during die-off), constipation, and irritable bowel symptoms disappeared very soon. Then the allergies began to lessen. The color returned to my face, and hair that had fallen out was replaced with new growth. After several months, I found that I had improved not only physically but mentally and emotionally, as well. Even though Vicki kept reminding me I wasn't totally well, my energy level would beg to differ! I began to feel like I was twenty years old again — happy, full of energy and hope for the future.

But the most important benefits of the 3-C Program for me were the dramatic changes in my cancer condition. In the beginning of this program, I would return to my cancer specialist every three weeks for blood testing that would inform us if the cancer had moved into my lymphatic system. Can you imagine how frightened and apprehensive I became with each visit, wondering if the cancer had spread? As I continued on the 3-C Program, my physical improvements were noticeable to everyone. My blood tests were looking better and better! Initially, my oncologist tried to be supportive of my lifestyle changes but admitted he was very skeptical. However, after my cancer went into total remission, he became very positive about the 3-C Program.

Three years later, my cancer is still in remission and none of my other symptoms have returned. I eat a healthy diet and am happy to say I can go anywhere I want and do anything I want. And best of all, I just had my first baby at 34 years of age after not being able to conceive for years. I have a healthy, beautiful boy who grew strong inside of me on a nutritious, vegetarian diet and will remain on one. He is a wonderful blessing, and I am thankful I learned how to be well; otherwise, he would never have been conceived. I have a great zest for life, a happy mental and emotional attitude, I look ten years younger than my age, and I think life is fantastic again!

Sue

Years ago, my thyroid was removed due to cancer. I also suffered from Candida, asthma, fibromyelitis (muscle and joint weakness and pain), arthritis, severe sinus and gall bladder condition, constipation, frequent and uncontrolled urination, severe environmental and food allergies, swollen throat, lymph glands and hands and feet, red face, blood-shot eyes, a constant metallic taste, and lack of appetite.

The chemical and environmental allergies were a major problem for me. In fact, my husband and I had to move 50 miles out of the city to an isolated, rural area so that I would not suffer from the chemical effects of modern society. Even here, I reacted to many different elements in my home as well as outside. I was so sensitive to cigarette smoke and burning fires that one exposure would affect me for weeks. Even the exhaust from a lawn mower or garden tiller could be detected from one-half mile away. I had to close all the doors and windows until the machinery was turned off. I lived on *Alka-Seltzer Gold*, which I realize now only added to my problem.

It is hard to imagine just how weak I was. I could not even open a door. After being diagnosed with Candida, I was put on nystatin and a high-protein, low-carbohydrate diet for sixteen months. Although I did make some improvement by being able to weight-lift 7 pounds, the improvement did not last long. I had to decrease the number of repetitions I weight-lifted and would lose an average of 3 pounds each time I did this. Also, I had difficulty with all of my joints. They would "give out" to the point where I could not even go up a flight of stairs. It would take months to regain my strength.

Even though the 3-C Program sounded promising, I was skeptical that I would be able to exercise for a full hour each morning. In the past, any attempt to exercise exhausted me to the point that I would simply end up in bed. After two weeks on the 3-C Program, I was amazed to find that I could walk for one hour, plus work a full day in my woodworking shop at home. I had not been able to do that for five years! After two months on the program, I could walk six miles; after four months, I could walk 13 miles; and after 7 months, I climbed Mt. La Conte in Tennessee. This mountain is 4,000 feet high, and climbing it involves a 15-mile hike. Also, after eight months, I was delighted to find that I could do several series of weight-lifting, using 15-pounds, without losing weight.

Much to my delight, after only a few weeks on this program, most of my chemical allergies disappeared. I am still amazed that I can now walk by a running lawn mower with no problem! Only cigarette smoke and burning fires still cause a slight reaction, and it lasts only a few hours. This is wonderful compared to my previous reactions that lasted several weeks. I can even travel with my husband again.

I have learned a lot from this program. I understand how to care for my body by providing it with the best of food, proper rest, reasonable exercise, and a positive attitude. After so many unsuccessful diets, procedures, and therapies, I am grateful the 3-C Program has enabled me to rejoin society!

Beth W.

Many women suffer the agonies of premenstrual syndrome, but for me this condition seemed totally beyond endurance. My symptoms became even more severe after the birth of my second child. I was nervous and anxious most of the time for no apparent reason. I had bouts of depression, spaciness, and incoordination, frequently just before my menstrual period. In addition, I noticed that even one alcoholic drink would cause depression and emotional instability for several days. An especially frustrating problem was scaly skin on my hands and fungus on my nails, which had been a problem since high school. Dermatologists had not been successful in treating this condition.

Suspecting Candida as my problem, my doctor put me on a typical high- protein, low-carbohydrate Candida recovery diet and nystatin, as well as a variety of supplements. However, it was necessary for me to discontinue taking nystatin due to adverse side effects, such as feeling like I was going crazy and crying all day long. Discouraged, I sought a second opinion. Through the use of a blood test, the second doctor also confirmed a Candida condition but was not able to offer a treatment of significant difference. Continued adherence to the diet caused me to lose 20 pounds on an already-slender frame. I heard of Vicki's experience and contacted her. After she described the principles of the 3-C Program, I decided it made sense and agreed to give it a try. Within a few months, my Candida and premenstrual problems were gone. So were the symptoms of anxiety, depression, and emotional ups and downs. My blood sugar stabilized, I had plenty of energy, and I looked forward to beginning each day. I enjoyed the recommended diet so much that I do not plan to alter it, Candida or no Candida.

Beth M.

Although things began to worsen when I was pregnant with my first child, I believe that my illness developed over a period of years beginning with my college days of junk food, alcohol, and stress. My symptoms were not severe and developed so gradually that I felt they were just things I would have to "put up with," although I continued to search for answers. My symptoms included Candida, low blood sugar, irritability, constant hunger, chronic fatigue, acne, split and weak nails, spaciness, PMS, lack of organization, low self- esteem, confusion, and depression. My daughter also displayed extreme irritability and hunger. She needed to be entertained most of the time.

After starting on the 3-C Program, I noticed these improvements: My acne and premenstrual syndrome disappeared, my nails are healthier-looking than ever before, and I can eat only two meals a day with no hunger symptoms. An added benefit was starting my daughter on this program at the same time. Even though not as sick as I, she has benefited greatly. Our irritability subsided drastically and continued to improve on a daily basis. Soon my daughter was playing by herself much of the time again. I no longer felt constantly tired and found that, for the first time, I could function from 5:00 AM until 9:00 PM at high energy levels. My house is organized and tidy because I now have the energy to keep it this way. Since I am no longer depressed, I have confidence that I never had before. It seems that, along with my house, my brain became organized as well!

I am so thankful for Vicki's help and for the knowledge I have gained through the 3-C Program. Words cannot describe how appreciative my family and I are. Feeling wonderful makes life fun again!

Ann Claire

Ann Claire, age 7, had a medical history that pointed directly at Candida as a factor in her numerous health problems. She suffered with repeated ear infections, postnasal drip, and enlarged tonsils. Even after surgery to remove her tonsils and adenoids at age 5, the ear infections, constant hacking cough, and sniffling continued. Her voice was hoarse and husky from the build-up of mucous, and she had rashes on her buttocks and painful irritation of the genital area. Wetting the bed had also become a problem.

Because her nasal passages were still congested following surgery, the doctor suspected allergies and sent her to be tested for food and environmental sensitivities. Test results indicated that she was allergic to a great many foods and environmental elements, including *Candida albicans*. She was given a strict diet, nystatin, several nutritional supplements, and desensitizing drops to be taken under the tongue. The nystatin medication caused side effects such as temper tantrums, uncontrolled bowel movements, and restless sleep. Therefore, it was discontinued after ten days.

After hearing about the 3-C Program, Ann Claire's mother contacted Vicki and started her on it immediately. All of her symptoms have been alleviated with the exception of occasional bed-wetting. Ann Claire has continued to remain well for several years.

Elizabeth

Elizabeth's health problems began at birth with a closed tear duct. She had daily drops of antibiotics in her eyes the entire first year of her life, and she also suffered repeated ear infections for which she was given numerous antibiotics until the age of three. In addition to severe rashes on her buttocks and painful irritation around the anal opening, she suffered several seizures before she was two years old. At the age of two and one half years, it was recommended that she be given the drug *Tegretol*, to control seizures. This was administered only for one week due to unfavorable side effects.

Elizabeth was seen by a specialist dealing in food and environmental sensitivities and was diagnosed as having Candida as well as multiple allergies. Nystatin was prescribed in addition to a typical Candida diet. Because of side effects such as temper tantrums, toilet problems, and nightmares, dosages of nystatin were discontinued.

In searching for an alternate treatment method, Elizabeth's family discovered the 3-C Program. Elizabeth began this program well over three years ago and we are very impressed with her progress. Her behavior has improved, she rarely wets the bed, and all other symptoms are relieved. We are especially thankful for the absence of ear infections and seizures.

Lauren

Lauren's health problems started immediately after her birth, including excessive amounts of chest mucous, bad stomachaches, and thrush. She manifested chest wheezing at 6-8 weeks. Chest X-rays revealed minute aspiration (fluid in the lungs). Other symptoms were frequent colds, ear infections, stomach problems, and bowel movements with extreme odor. At 9 months, Lauren developed asthma complicated by pneumonia, bronchitis, unexplained fevers and rashes. She would have periods of screaming and crying for up to two hours. By ten months of age, additional symptoms included severe rectal gas, eye swelling, and rashes on her buttocks that caused her skin to peel. She was hospitalized for the pneumonia and had tubes inserted into her ears. When questioned about the frequency of her illness, Lauren's doctor said that she had an "immature immune system" and would grow out of it. During this period, she was treated with many antibiotics and cortisone.

At eighteen months of age, Lauren began seeing a clinical ecologist/allergist who started treatment with allergy extract injections and a rotation diet. Lauren improved for seven months but quickly and mysteriously began to deteriorate again. Respiratory, behavioral, and gas problems multiplied. She developed a severe vaginal itch that would often produce a green discharge and caused extreme pain. Having exhausted all other means, the allergist contacted Dr. William Crook and started Lauren on a yeast-free diet, supplemented with nystatin. Lauren was allergic to all vitamin and mineral supplements. She improved slightly, but the symptoms still continued. Up to this point, Lauren's mother calculated they had spent in excess of $20,000 on doctors, hospitals, medicines, tests, cotton mattresses, and other miscellaneous expenses.

Lauren's mother contacted Vicki and subsequently started Lauren on the 3-C Program, which involved the use of whole foods in a vegetarian format, plus the use of a liquid garlic concentrate to rebuild the immune system. After two weeks on this program, Lauren's condition improved dramatically. She stopped her allergy shots and nystatin medication. Within one month, all itching, respiratory, and bowel symptoms cleared up, and her behavior was much improved. She did have some bad days initially as the yeast was being reduced but continued to make steady improvement. Lauren has not had to visit doctors, take medication, or be hospitalized since starting the 3-C Program over three years ago. Quite an accomplishment for such a sick little girl!

CHAPTER 2
THE CANDIDA CULPRIT

WHAT IS CANDIDA?

There are hundreds of different types of microorganisms, or germs, that live in and on the human body, such as bacteria and fungi (yeast). *Candida albicans* (hereafter referred to as "Candida" or "yeast") is the name of a particularly hardy type of yeast microorganism that belongs to the family of molds, mildew and fungi (much like a zucchini is a variety of squash in the vegetable family). Candida is normally found in the digestive tract starting at the mouth and ending at the rectum and/or the urinary tract and male/female genitals.

Also found in the digestive tract are bacterial microorganisms, which differ from yeast microorganisms. One type of bacteria, called *lactobacillus acidophilus*, forms a natural flora, or balance, between these two families of microorganisms. The *lactobacillus acidophilus* are the "good guys," or friendly bacteria.

In a healthy individual, the good bacteria greatly outnumber the yeast microorganisms, thereby keeping the yeast from multiplying and feeding off of the body like a parasite does. As long as this balance is maintained, the yeasts are not capable of causing disease. However, if the good bacteria are destroyed, there is nothing to keep the yeast under control. They are now able to grow out of control, functioning as "bad guys" in the body.

Destruction of good bacteria can be attributed to many circumstances, including nutritional deficiencies, hormonal changes during pregnancy or menstrual cycles, and the use of antibiotics or hormone/steroid-based compounds. Many people today are consuming hormones often unknowingly through the use of birth control pills, anti-inflammatory medications, or in estrogen-replacement therapy. In the past decade these various compounds have been prescribed in much larger quantities than ever before.

With a reduced amount of good bacteria in the body, combined with a diet high in yeast products and sugar, yeast organisms can multiply at an even greater rate. While localized yeast symptoms can appear in the form of a vaginal infection, thrush or in some organs, yeast organisms can also change from a simple yeast to an invasive fungus. The result is a condition called "polysystemic chronic Candidiasis," meaning yeast or fungal toxins affecting the entire system. One of the most potent toxins emitted by yeast is acetaldehyde, which is similar to formaldehyde (embalming fluid)!

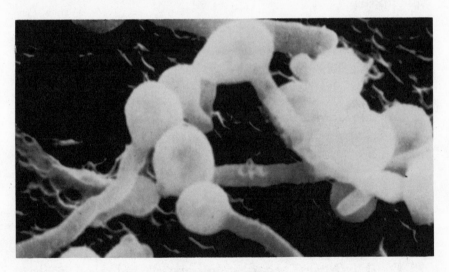

Candida albicans

This electron microscope photograph of *Candida albicans* in the human gut, is magnified 1,000,000 times. Note the feeding tubes called *hyphae* seeking nourishment from its human victim. During this growth process, toxic materials are emitted, which spread through the body to produce various Candida symptoms.

POSSIBLE SYMPTOMS OF CANDIDA

Listed below are some of the more common Candida symptoms:

General Symptoms: Loss of appetite or cravings for certain foods or drinks, fatigue, loss of hair, weight gain or loss, incoordination or dizziness, insomnia or lethargy. Symptoms may be worse on damp days or when around damp or moldy areas.

Emotional Symptoms: Feeling "out in left field," "spaced out," nervous, anxious, depressed, confused, or experiencing poor memory. Having mood swings, headaches, or hypoglycemic-like symptoms, even though test results may not be conclusive.

Stomach/Intestinal Symptoms: Indigestion, gas, bloating, belching, diarrhea, constipation, colitis, Crohn's Disease, irritable bowel syndrome, spastic colon, gastritis, mucous in stool, rectal itching, or hemorrhoids.

Cardiovascular Symptoms: Poor circulation, tightness in chest, asthma, wheezing, coughing, or mitral valve prolapse.

Muscle/Joint Symptoms: Numbness, paralysis or tingling of the extremities, poor coordination, weakness, aches and pains of joints or muscles, stiffness, swelling, or arthritis.

Urinary Symptoms: Burning, frequent infections of the kidney or bladder, or frequent urinating.

Eye/Ear/Nose/Throat Symptoms: Blurred vision, spots in front of eyes, eye or ear infections, pain or fluid in ears, deafness or sensitivity to noise, gum problems, white patches in mouth (especially on the tongue), coughing, bad breath, nasal congestion, postnasal drip, or sinus problems.

Skin Symptoms: Acne, itching, dryness or oiliness, scaly skin or psoriasis, athlete's foot, toenail or fingernail fungus, soreness, or ridges in nails.

Allergic Symptoms: Rashes, itching, hives, asthma, hay fever, or food or chemical sensitivities.

Additional Symptoms Specific To Women: Vaginal discharge, itching, burning, PMS or menstrual cycle abnormalities, endometriosis, or sexual dysfunction.

Additional Symptoms Specific To Men: Loss of sexual vigor, prostate problems, or impotence.

Additional Symptoms Usually Specific To Children: Thrush, diaper rash, colic, recurring ear infections, hyperactivity, learning difficulties, short attention span, nasal congestion, coughing, digestive problems, or cravings for certain foods, usually sweets.

Anyone can appreciate by reviewing these possible symptoms that Candida contributes to many chronic illnesses. Naturally, just because a person experiences one or more of these symptoms does not necessarily mean he or she has Candida. On the other hand, a person who does have Candida may experience either just a few or many of these symptoms.

Some health professionals feel certain blood tests are valuable in helping to diagnose Candida-related illnesses. Others rely heavily on an individual's symptoms. Below is an abbreviated questionnaire to better determine whether Candida is a possibility in one's health problems.

CANDIDA ILLNESS QUESTIONNAIRE

Answer each question "YES" or "NO" by making a check mark in the appropriate column.

PART I — MEDICAL HISTORY

A. Have you had (or do you now have)
1. Thyroid treatments? . . . . Yes   No
2. Diabetes?   . . . . Yes   No
3. Cancer in any form? . . . . Yes   No
4. Hypoglycemia? . . . . Yes   No

B. Have you had:
1. Operation(s)?   . . . . Yes   No
2. Catheterization(s)? . . . . Yes   No
3. Anti-cancer medication(s)? . . . . Yes   No
4. Radiation treatment(s)? . . . . Yes   No

C. Have you taken:
1. Antibiotics? . . . . Yes   No
2. Tetracycline for acne? . . . . Yes   No
3. Oral contraceptives? . . . . Yes   No
4. Oral or injected cortisone? (includes Prednisone) . . . . Yes   No

D. Do you live (or have you lived) in a:
1. Damp climate? . . . . Yes   No
2. Moldy house? . . . . Yes   No
3. Area of foggy beaches? . . . . Yes   No

E. Do you have (or have you ever had)
1. an alcohol problem? . . . . Yes   No

F. Do you use (or have you ever used)
1. Marijuana? . . . . Yes   No
2. Cocaine? . . . . Yes   No
3. Heroin? . . . . Yes   No

G. Have you had recurrent viral or bacterial infections? . Yes   No

H. Have you had recurrent yeast infections?
1. Vaginal . . . . Yes   No
2. Nail . . . . Yes   No
3. Thrush . . . . Yes   No
4. Jock itch . . . . Yes   No

PART II — PRESENT SITUATION

A. Are your symptoms worse
1. When raking dry leaves? . . . . Yes   No
2. In a damp basement? . . . . Yes   No
3. On rainy or humid days? . . . . Yes   No

B. Do you crave
1. Sugar? . . . . Yes   No

2. Breads? . . . . Yes   No
3. Milk products? . . . . Yes   No
4. Alcohol? . . . . Yes   No

C. Are you uncomfortable when in contact with
1. Smoke (any type)? . . . . Yes   No
2. Fumes (any type)? . . . . Yes   No
3. Agricultural chemicals? . . . . Yes   No
4. Perfume, cologne, soaps, laundry detergent? . . . . . . Yes   No

PART III — DIGESTIVE SYSTEM SYMPTOMS
Are the following symptoms present?
1. Gas/Abdominal distension . . . . Yes   No
2. Diarrhea/Constipation . . . . Yes   No
3. Hemorrhoids . . . . Yes   No
4. Anal itching . . . . Yes   No
5. Mucus in stools . . . . Yes   No
6. Heartburn/Indigestion . . . . Yes   No
7. Bad breath . . . . Yes   No
8. Constant hunger feeling . . . . Yes   No
9. Food allergies . . . . Yes   No
10. Weight gain/loss without change in diet . . . . Yes   No
11. Thick white/yellow coating on tongue in morning . . . . Yes   No

PART IV — MENTAL/HEAD SYMPTOMS
Are the following symptoms present?
1. Difficulty in concentration . . . . Yes   No
2. Short attention span . . . . Yes   No
3. Memory retention difficulty . . . . Yes   No
4. Fogginess, spaciness . . . . Yes   No
5. Excessive sleepiness . . . . Yes   No
6. Headaches . . . . Yes   No
7. Depression and/or suicidal thoughts . . . . Yes   No
8. Mood swings . . . . Yes   No
9. Irritability/Anger/Confusion . . . . Yes   No

PART V — HORMONAL SYMPTOMS
1. Are the following symptoms present? . . . . Yes   No
2. Premenstrual syndrome . . . . Yes   No
3. Yeast infection week before period . . . . Yes   No
4. Decreased sexual desire . . . . Yes   No
5. Impotence . . . . Yes   No
6. Endometriosis . . . . Yes   No
7. Menstrual irregularities . . . . Yes   No
8. Yeast infection after intercourse . . . . Yes   No

PART VI — MISCELLANEOUS SYMPTOMS
Are the following symptoms present?
1. Tightness in chest . . . . Yes   No

2. Heart palpitations . . . . Yes   No
3. Urinary frequency, urgency, burning . . . . Yes   No
4. Post nasal drip . . . . Yes   No
5. Muscle/joint pains . . . . Yes   No
6. Incoordination, balance problems . . . . Yes   No
7. Cold hands/feet . . . . Yes   No
8. Water retention (Edema) . . . . Yes   No
9. Prostatitis . . . . Yes   No
10. Swallowing difficulties/Sore throat . . . . Yes   No
11. Eyes burning, tearing . . . . Yes   No
12. Itching, scaling skin . . . . Yes   No

TOTAL POSSIBLE 'YES' ANSWERS IS 75.

YOUR SCORE: _____

Guidelines:

If score is 50 or more yes answers, a Candida-related illness is very likely.

If score is 40 or more yes answers, a Candida-related illness is probably a factor.

If score is 30 or more yes answers, a Candida-related illness is possible.

Candida Testing

There are several tests available that attempt to determine if a person may have Candida overgrowth, along with much controversy as to their reliability. Some health professionals feel that these tests only confirm that even healthy people have a certain amount of Candida in their body, with resultant antibodies. Other professionals value the results of these tests as another factor in determining if a Candida-related illness is a possibility.

The author was tested using the IgA, IgM, and IgG Candida Antibody Test. Through blood samples, this test measures the levels of A antibodies (those secreted by mucous membranes), M antibodies (which are the first antibodies produced in response to foreign invaders), and G antibodies (long-term antibodies produced by B-cell lymphocytes). Four months after initiating the 3-C Program, the author was retested using the same procedure and the same laboratory, and results showed that her yeast level had dropped to a normal range.

As previously mentioned, there are many different types of yeast organisms in human bodies. Although *Candida albicans* is the most common, it is possible to have an overgrowth of a strain other than or in addition to *Candida albicans*, such as *Candida tropicalis* or *Candida parapsilosis*. Keep in mind that typical yeast blood tests are formulated to detect the *Candida albicans* strain specifically. If a blood test shows a normal or low amount of *Candida albicans*, further testing may be necessary to detect the possibility of overgrowth of a less common yeast strain. Testing for a strain of yeast other than *Candida albicans* can be more costly, and this service is often not available. The 3-C Program does, however, address all types of yeast infections.

There is an excellent book by Dr. William Crook titled *The Yeast Connection*. Dr. Crook is a wonderful physician who studied the findings of Dr. Orian Truss and has made great progress in bringing Candida-related illness to the attention of the medical community as well as the public. His book, and others listed in the Reference section in this book, will provide more in-depth information and explanations concerning Candida. However, diet and other health principles recommended in Dr. Crook's book vary from those of the 3-C Program. For many people the "typical" Candida treatment program described in Dr. Crook's treatment program does provide sufficient relief. However, for others the level of improvement is not substantial enough to allow them to return to what they consider optimal health. For these people a strict vegetarian diet, along with an emphasis on alternative lifestyle choices (especially focusing on those that address the digestive system), is necessary in order to overcome their health problems. When implemented and followed carefully, the 3-C Program has experienced an exceptional success rate.

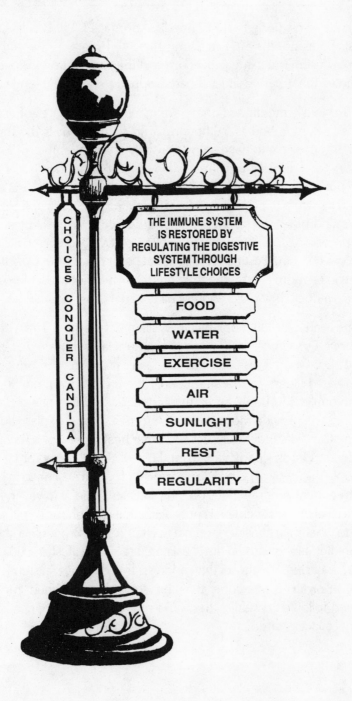

CHOICES CONQUER CANDIDA

THE IMMUNE SYSTEM IS RESTORED BY REGULATING THE DIGESTIVE SYSTEM THROUGH LIFESTYLE CHOICES

FOOD

WATER

EXERCISE

AIR

SUNLIGHT

REST

REGULARITY

CHAPTER 3

CHOICES CONQUER CANDIDA

THE 3-C CONCEPT

The program outlined in this book is called the "3-C Program," which stands for "Choices Conquer Candida." The concept behind this program is that making proper *lifestyle choices* that regulate the *digestive system* will in turn strengthen the *immune system*, thus eliminating yeast overgrowth. Because the elements that promote a yeast overgrowth are cumulative and may take many years to appear, few have examined the connection between lifestyle and Candida; instead they have typically only treated symptoms when they appear. Just as modern technology has changed, so have priorities and, consequently, lifestyle choices and habits. Subsequently, through no fault of their own, people have been making unwise lifestyle choices concerning the care and maintenance of their bodies for far too long. The 3-C Program addresses the condition of Candida, as well as other illnesses, by highlighting corrective lifestyle choices that have been proven to improve overall health.

There are many different theories available today concerning the treatment of Candida, and most of them address two common elements: first, reducing existing yeast overgrowth via the use of an anti-fungal preparation such as nystatin, and second, rebuilding the immune system through the use of supplements. While these programs have merit and do work for some, they are unsuccessful for many others. In their previous treatment programs, Candida patients may have noticed a degree of improvement at first, but then have regressed. Or, they may have reached a degree of improvement but never moved beyond that stage. They become quite desperate, wondering if there really is an answer. They don't know where to turn and feel like screaming every time they hear of another Candida treatment program. Some have banded together in support groups, working very hard to gather any and all helpful information regarding their condition. But they are still not well and are tired of sacrificing all or part of their lives to this devastating illness.

In successfully treating Candida, it is important to realize that *the deterioration of an immune system is never due to just one factor.* It is usually a slow, cumulative process due to many factors, including poor diet, excessive medications, use of tobacco and/or alcohol, and poor quality water, as well as a lack of exercise, fresh air, sunshine, and rest. In fact, it is a contradiction of terms to refer to typical habits as a "lifestyle." "Existence-style" might be more descriptive. Bad habits and poor lifestyle choices that conform to modern rat-race schedules are contradictory to the body's natural biological time clock. The care of the body becomes no longer a focus but an afterthought.

Degenerative illnesses attributed to poor lifestyle choices have an excellent chance of improvement and/or reversal. However, that is not to say that such health conditions as certain predisposed genetic conditions can be totally reverse due to lifestyle change. Dietary and other deficiencies and their resultant health problems may be passed down from one's ancestors. For example, if their diets were lacking in certain nutrients then it is more than likely their children will inherit the tendency toward health conditions resulting from that deficiency.

The good news is that proper lifestyle choices can strengthen the immune system so that it is not as vulnerable to inherited weaknesses. Remember, *it is possible to control the majority of factors that contribute to one's health* simply by learning the proper choices.

The 3-C Program is based on this concept: *The immune system is restored by regulating the digestive system through lifestyle choices which aid in reducing candida and other degenerative illness.*

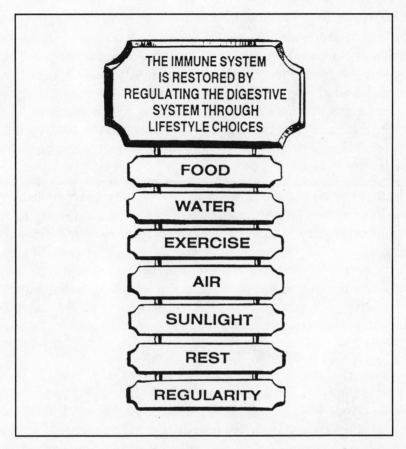

The 3-C Program differs from others in that the use of its principles begins to rebuild the immune system immediately. It will eliminate lifestyle choices that have been, unknowingly, contributing to illness and will replace them with those that promote healing and good health. As these choices are addressed in upcoming chapters, some of them may seem trivial at first glance. However, it is important to realize that they all fit together like pieces of a puzzle to promote healing and good health that will last a lifetime!

THE DIGESTIVE SYSTEM

Because the proper functioning of the digestive system is so crucial in Candida recovery, it is necessary to understand how the digestion process works. Digestion actually begins in the mouth where chewing breaks down large pieces of food into smaller ones. Salivary glands in the mouth produce saliva, which contains ptyalin, an enzyme that breaks down carbohydrates. Active chemical digestion begins in the stomach, where the food is mixed with hydrochloric acid, water, and enzymes, which begin to break down protein and other substances. After a certain number of hours, depending on the combination of foods, this liquid form of food (chyme) moves into the small intestine in the following order: carbohydrates, protein, and then fat, which takes the longest to digest.

In the small intestine, the pancreas secretes its digestive juices. An emulsifier called bile is secreted by the liver if fats are present in the food. The pancreas also secretes substances that neutralize the digestive acids and further help to break down proteins and carbohydrates so they can be absorbed. The remaining undigested products enter the large intestine and eventually are excreted. No digestive enzymes are secreted in the large intestine and little change occurs there except for the absorption of water.

Functioning properly, this very delicate process of digestion is a wonder of nature. However, if for any reason it is delayed, food will remain in the stomach longer than it should, putrefying and creating fermentation. Most people would never consider eating food that should normally be refrigerated but has been sitting at room temperature for hours because they understand it would eventually decay, ferment, and grow harmful bacteria. However, they are not aware that conditions in the stomach are even more perfect for this decaying process since the stomach is constantly dark, damp, and warmer than room temperature!

It is crucial for Candida patients to realize that this fermentation process produces not only unhealthy bacteria but, more notably, alcohol-like products! In fact, there is a strain of yeast reported from Japan that actually produces pure alcohol in the colon. These alcohol-like chemicals, such as aldehydes and esters, are toxic to the entire system, especially the brain, liver and kidneys. They can also be held accountable for a variety of symptoms common to many Candida patients, such as fatigue, spaciness, confusion, uncoordination, and depression. No wonder Candida patients actually experience mild intoxication!

Even though several authorities feel that it is technically inaccurate to use the term "feeding the yeast," many Candida patients identify this term with the use of certain foods or beverages that often cause an increase in their symptoms, such as alcohol, sugar, and other yeast products. Though these items do not directly "feed" yeast, their sugar and simple carbohydrate content very often cause sensitivities in Candida patients.

Just as it would not be wise to consume alcohol when battling a yeast overgrowth, it would also not be wise to allow the creation of it in the stomach by delaying the digestion process and causing fermentation. Yet this is exactly what happens when proper digestion principles are ignored. Digestion is delayed, which causes fermentation, producing alcohol-like products that, in addition to causing other symptoms, can *actually encourage more yeast growth!* Additionally, this fermentation process is a major source of intestinal gas and indigestion.

A major objective of the 3-C Program is to correct lifestyle choices that delay the digestion process, which causes fermentation and production of alcohol-like products that support yeast growth. Reference to any form of the word "delay" will appear in bold print throughout the rest of this book as a reminder of the connection between delaying the digestion process, Candida and poor health in general.

It is vital that the principles of digestion are understood. These principles will also help to emphasize the significance of other lifestyle choices discussed in upcoming chapters and how they also affect the digestive system.

Principles That Regulate The Digestive System:

1. Chew Food Well

Chewing food well should be more than simply something remembered from elementary school. Even though most people do not make the connection between chewing food and what goes on in their stomach, chewing food thoroughly is crucial to good digestion. *The first stage of digestion starts in the mouth.* The jaws and teeth provide the first mechanical breakdown of food. Unless food is chewed to a "cream" consistency, "chunks" of food will enter the stomach and will not be digested nearly as well as food thoroughly chewed. A **delay** in digestion could occur, resulting in gas and indigestion.

Saliva plays a major role in this first stage of digestion. Loaded with enzymes, saliva provides the initial chemical breakdown. Without the proper amount of saliva, there will be a shortage of enzymes to initiate the digestion process. Some suggestions for promoting good saliva production and facilitating good digestion are:

—Take small bites of food and chew to a cream consistency.

—Mealtimes should be relaxed.

—An average mealtime should last approximately 30 to 40 minutes. If it takes longer than this to eat, one can chew a little faster, but still thoroughly.

—Eliminate chewing gum. Chewing gum causes saliva to be secreted continuously, "using up" the enzymes it contains so necessary to digestion. Remember, as long as the jaw is moving, saliva is being produced and is being depleted. Chewing gum depletes the saliva supply that is needed at mealtimes.

—Have regular mealtimes. Eating at different times every day disrupts the rhythmical saliva response. However, eating at the same time every day insures that saliva production is more abundant and efficient.

—Drink enough water between meals to promote saliva production. Adequate water between meals makes certain there is abundant saliva available at mealtimes to help swallow food, thereby eliminating the need for liquids at mealtimes. (See #3 below.)

2. Eat Two Or Three Meals A Day With Nothing Between

Eating between meals is probably the *worst offender of proper digestion*, and it doesn't matter what or how much is eaten. Even as little as a peanut will **delay** stomach emptying and digestion — not by merely a few minutes but by many hours, as research cited below indicates.

In a study at the New England Sanitarium, a healthy nurse was given an ordinary breakfast at 7:30 AM along with barium, a substance used in tracing the stomach's digestion. She ate a piece of fudge four times throughout the day, at 9:00 AM, 11:00 AM, 2:00 PM, and 4:00 PM. This nurse also ate dinner at 12:00 noon and supper at 6:00 PM. X-rays revealed that one-half of her breakfast was still in her stomach at 9:30 that evening!

Studies at Loma Linda University have confirmed the same facts. Students given a routine breakfast of cereal with cream, bread, cooked fruit, and an egg were found to have emptied their stomachs within 4 to 5 hours. Several days later, these same students were given the same breakfast. However, some time later they consumed various snacks. The chart below shows what snacks each student consumed and for how many hours these snacks extended the time their original breakfast remained in their stomachs.

NORMAL BREAKFAST	FOOD EATEN LATER	BREAKFAST RESIDUE STILL IN STOMACH
Student #1	Ice cream cone (2 hours later)	After 6 hours
Student #2	Peanut butter sandwich (2 hours later)	After 9 hours
Student #3	Pumpkin pie & milk (2 hours later)	After 9 hours
Student #4	1/2 slice bread & butter (every 90 minutes but no dinner)	Over half of meal after 9 hours
Student #5	.A little bit of chocolate twice in AM and twice in PM	13 and 1/2 hours later more than one half of breakfast still in stomach

As can be seen, the common practice of eating too often causes food to sit in the stomach for hours longer than it should. That's why it is essential to *wait at least 5 hours from the end of one meal to the beginning of the next meal* so that there is ample time for the stomach to empty. Even after recovery, it is best to leave five hours between meals. At the very least, four and one-half hours would be acceptable.

3. Liquids Should Not Be Consumed With Meals

Drinking any liquids (even water) with meals, or consuming too much of the liquids used in cooking foods such as soups or stews very definitely **delays** digestion for several reasons. First, natural enzymes contained in human saliva are vital in breaking down food. Liquids actually dilute and weaken these enzymes, resulting in less efficient digestion. Second, the stomach must maintain an important acid/alkaline balance in order to do its job properly. Extra liquid in the stomach upsets this balance, also **delaying** the digestion process. Third, most liquids consumed with meals are either very hot or very cold, causing a **delay** in digestion while the stomach works to regulate everything to a more normal temperature. (This same stress results from eating foods that are either very hot or cold.)

The need to drink liquids with meals to help "wash" down food can most often be attributed to insufficient water *between* meals. As stated earlier, adequate water between meals produces more abundant amounts of saliva that aid in the chewing and swallowing process, in addition to eliminating a feeling of thirst.

4. Eliminate Eating In The Evenings

Another detrimental, yet common, lifestyle habit is eating in the evenings, whether it be snacking or late meals. Ideally, the digestive system should function like the rest of the body, alert and energetic. Research shows that calories are more quickly and efficiently burned *early* in the day, demonstrating the fact that the digestive system is also more efficient early in the day. (This is particularly noteworthy if trying to lose weight.)

As the day progresses, energy sources become depleted, mentally and physically. Just as a person feels "worn out," so does her (or his) digestive system, especially after breaking down two or three meals. Imagine how it feels after attempting to digest five or six! Eating late in the evening is like asking the digestive system to work "second shift" after just completing first shift. The feeling is similar to how one would feel after staying up all night. Constantly eating late at night puts a burden on the entire digestive system and other organs because the entire digestion process starts all over again *every time something is eaten, no matter what or how much.* Just as the rest of the body benefits from rest, the digestive system needs to heal and rejuvenate at night.

An added burden from eating late at night occurs because of lying down. Reclining after meals or going to bed after a snack causes food to empty less efficiently from the stomach because the weight of the stomach compresses large nerves on either side of the spinal column. This action shuts off the mechanism that keeps the digestive process working. Therefore, both eating in the evenings and reclining after eating will **delay** digestion. If one chooses to follow the three-meal plan of the 3-C Program rather than the preferred two-meal plan, she (or he) should be certain to leave at least three hours between the third meal and bedtime. (See Chapter 5, Getting Well.) This optional third meal should be the smallest, simplest meal of the day, equalling no more than 10 to 20 percent of daily food intake.

5. Reduce The Number Of Foods At Each Meal

Eating in a restaurant today brings to mind how many different items are included in a typical meal. For example, if a meal were to include meat, several kinds of vegetables, bread, butter, a beverage, salad or salad bar (anywhere from four to ten additional items), it would require the digestive system to break down anywhere from ten to twenty different foods! Since each food has a different molecular structure, requiring enzymes, energy, and time for dismantling, no wonder eating too many varieties at a meal can overwhelm the stomach. Too many different foods creates "competition" for enzymes. They are not able to effectively break down all the various foods, which results in **delay** in digestion.

Unfortunately, when the digestive system suffers, the whole body suffers. Since the digestion process does require body energy to complete, it would be less taxing on the entire body if a smaller variety of foods was consumed at each meal. Historic indications lead one to believe that our early ancestors ate only one food at a meal. Though primitive, they must have followed their bodies' natural instinct. In contrast, mealtime is now a product of modern society, with an effort to "have it all."

For these reasons, no more than three or four different foods should be consumed at one meal until one has recovered. If a person has severe digestion or other health problems, three items would be best. Otherwise, four items are good to start with, moving up to five once one has recovered. (Counting items at a meal will be discussed in Chapter 8.)

6. Practice Simple Food Combining

The 3-C Program is not a heavily restrictive food-combining program. There are two basic food combining guidelines: Fruits and vegetables should not be combined at the same meal, and vegetables should not be eaten at the third meal of the day.

Fruits and vegetables consist of different chemical compositions that compete with each other for absorption, causing **delay** in the digestion process. Combining these two food groups can cause gas, indigestion, and a decrease in vitamin absorption. Fruits are much easier to digest than vegetables; therefore, vegetables should not be

SIMPLE FOOD COMBINING

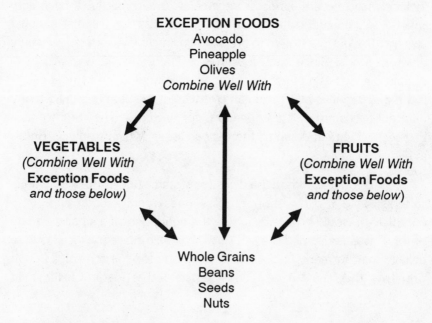

EXCEPTION FOODS
Avocado
Pineapple
Olives
Combine Well With

VEGETABLES
(Combine Well With
Exception Foods
and those below)

FRUITS
(Combine Well With
Exception Foods
and those below)

Whole Grains
Beans
Seeds
Nuts

eaten at the third meal. Very simply put, vegetables can be eaten with any food group except fruit. Likewise, fruit can be eaten with any food group except vegetables.

7. Limit Refined And Concentrated Foods

Avoiding concentrated and refined foods is a key element in the 3-C Program. Concentrated foods have been taken out of their natural state and condensed into another product. A common example is an orange, which is more often consumed in concentrated form (as a beverage) rather than in its whole state. Depending on the size and variety of the orange, it could take between four and eight oranges to make one glass of orange juice! Drinking a concentrated amount of these nutrients without the beneficial fiber and pulp causes orange juice to react differently in the body than if eating the whole orange.

In addition to being taken out of their natural state, refined foods also have the added insult of being recombined in another form. A seriously over-used refined food today is fat. Fat is often considered as to how saturated and unsaturated it is. Although there are some exceptions, saturated fats are solid at room temperature and are from animal sources. Unsaturated fats are mostly liquids (oils) from plant sources. The chart illustrates that unsaturated fats are further divided into categories of monounsaturated and polyunsaturated

A FEW FOODS HIGH IN SATURATED FAT

Beef	Cheese	Chocolate
Veal	Butter	Lard
Chicken	Milk	Coconut Oil
Pork	Cream	Palm Oil

A FEW FOODS HIGH IN UNSATURATED FAT

Polyunsaturates	Monounsaturates
Corn Oil	Peanut Oil
Safflower Oil	Cottonseed Oil
Soybean Oil	Olive Oil
Sesame Oil	Almonds
Mayonnaise	Peanuts
Soft Margarine	Avocados

In an effort to reduce heart disease, many people have been advised to substitute unsaturated fat for saturated fat. Even though unsaturated fats are supposedly better than saturated fats, they are still a concentrated product. For instance, it takes an average of 12 to 14 medium-sized ears of corn to equal one tablespoon of corn oil! Realistically, a typical meal could include not only one tablespoon of oil, but many. In fact, a survey of a meal eaten at a fast food salad bar that consisted of pasta with sauce, beans, rice, corn chips, and salad with dressing equalled nearly one-half cup of oil! Fats of some kind appear in nearly all packaged and processed foods, including cake mixes, cookies, muffins, crackers, and frozen and canned goods. Worse yet is the *amount* of fat used in products. Fats quite often appear as the second or third ingredient on package labels, meaning that fat content is nearly as much as the main ingredient. Food manufacturers benefit from adding fats to food because they are inexpensive, tasty, and give food products an appealing consistency.

Processed fats pose several health threats. Numerous processing techniques involving high heat and chemicals are required to produce a clear, tasteless fat product such as oil. Not only are precious vitamins and minerals destroyed but rancidity is very likely, causing free radical formation, which promotes cancer.

Free radical formation is difficult to explain in a few words but, stated very simply, free radicals are certain atoms that are highly reactive because of the way their electrons behave. Although a small number of free radicals is not dangerous, several factors can promote increased formation, which can have devastating effects on the cells of the body. One of these factors is consuming refined fats.

Even though everyone needs to consume a little fat for nutritional purposes, *whole foods* containing fat also contain vitamins and minerals that act as antioxidants to prevent free radical formation. Refined fats, however, have lost these precious nutrients and additionally may be rancid — both contributing to free radical formation. No wonder fats are referred to as "empty calories."

Fats also tends to "thicken" the cells of the body, discouraging maximum absorption of nutrients. Combined with a low-fiber diet and lack of exercise, there is little to combat this process. It is not surprising that refined fats have been associated with degenerative diseases such as accelerated aging, heart disease and more recently, cancer.

Although it is always preferable to eat foods in their whole, natural state, a good rule of thumb to follow when using a refined or concentrated product is *to limit the amount to no more than what could be consumed of that food in its whole state at one meal.*

8. Proper Exercise At Proper Times

Even though most people realize exercise is beneficial, very few are aware that *when* a person exercises has an impact on the digestive process. While the 3-C Program encourages exercise, strenuous activity immediately before or after a meal can **delay** the digestion process. Therefore, it would be better to perform fast-paced or strenuous forms of exercise, such as jogging, on an empty or near-empty stomach. On the other hand, mild exercise, such as light housework, gardening, or shopping, actually promotes moving food out of the stomach and into the other digestive organs.

9. Control Stress

An old adage, "One should never eat when upset," has, unfortunately, been more ignored than observed. Stress can have a definite affect on normal enzyme production, causing less absorption of nutrients and **delay** in the digestion process. It is better to skip a meal entirely, possibly having a cup of hot water with lemon juice or just a glass of water. After recovery, a cup of a simple herb tea would probably be well-tolerated. (See section on herb teas, Chapter 4, Water.)

SUMMARY

The digestive system is like a fine piece of mechanical equipment that begins to "bog down" under the weight of burdensome refined and concentrated foods. However, even if one is eating a good diet, certain habits and practices that disrupt the regular, rhythmical cycle of digestion can render a digestive system that has a difficult time effectively absorbing nutrients from food or supplements. Perhaps this is why some Candida patients struggle to recover, in spite of a good diet and supplements. Even in the absence of Candida overgrowth, a poorly functioning digestive system can promote other maladies such as gas, indigestion, allergies, lack of energy, insomnia or restless sleep, and fatigue. Added to other poor lifestyle choices, these inconvenient symptoms can escalate into major illness.

PRINCIPLES THAT REGULATE THE DIGESTIVE SYSTEM

Chew Food Well
Eat Two Or Three Meals A Day With Nothing Between
Liquids Should Not Be Consumed With Meals
Eliminate Eating In The Evenings
Reduce Number Of Foods At Each Meal
Practice Simple Food Combining
Limit Refined And Concentrated Foods
Utilize Proper Exercise At Proper Times
Control Stress

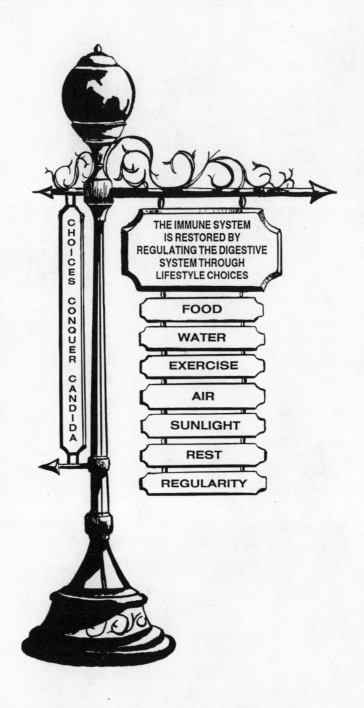

CHAPTER 4
LIFESTYLE CHOICES AND HEALTH

In order to gain a better understanding of proper care of the body, consider this analogy. If a fish is taken out of water and placed on dry ground, how long would it struggle before it becomes still? Or, if it is left in the water and the water is tainted with chemicals, heavy metals, and raw sewage, how long would it last? Or, if the fish is kept in fairly clean water, but given a very poor grade of nutrients, how long before sluggishness would set in, and then stillness?

A similar experiment can be performed with a non-feeling, non-caring automobile. If it were driven all winter on northern roads behind the salt spreader, then taken to the beach for the summer, and if molasses was used in place of motor oil (they both look the same), how would the car perform? No need to worry about the water in the radiator, after all, an optimist would say "it's half full, not half empty." And the kind of gas that goes into the tank makes absolutely no difference; after all, gas is gas, right? And instead of shutting the engine off each time it is parked, just let it run continuously and see what falls apart first, and how long it takes.

Since this is a book about health care and not fish husbandry or car care, the application of these two scenarios should be obvious. Great concern is placed upon animals and wildlife in modern society; likewise, cars are pampered like the major investment they are. Yet, with all of our humanitarian and economic interests, we fail to maintain the most valuable and complex of all machines: the human body. It is exposed to, filled with, burdened under, and demanded from more than good human reasoning should allow, and it is done day after day, year after year. There are many lifestyle choices that affect health, just as a multitude of factors affect fish or Fords. What is put into the body and what the body is exposed to demands far more attention than has typically been given. Many of these factors and how they can affect recovery from Candida, as well as other illness, are addressed in this chapter.

FOOD/*3-C PRINCIPLE*

Although the phrase, "garbage in, garbage out" has been used concerning many different subjects, it is especially true when it applies to the human diet. The bottom line is that poor diet equals poor health! Why is there not enough emphasis placed on the connection between good health and good food? Perhaps it is because of a wide-spread misunderstanding of what constitutes a healthy diet. About a century ago, the food in typical diets was less processed, less refined, and naturally more nutritious than the foods readily available today. Unfortunately, no one is pointing this out today because many health professionals do not make the connection between poor health and poor diet. Nutritional education is not a number-one priority in medical school. Time is devoted to the *treatment* of disease rather than the *prevention* of it.

If a doctor doesn't realize that refined, packaged, artificial, and chemical-laden foods should be avoided, how can that doctor pass this information on to patients? How many times, when symptoms of poor health cannot be accounted for, are the issues of food quality and water quality addressed? Hardly ever! Doctors seldom focus on the subjects of diet and nutrition and further complicate the issue by prescribing medications to cope with chronic ailments. When these medications fail to work, it is not uncommon for a person to be told they will "just have to live with it." It's no wonder that, even though modern medicine has conquered some diseases, degenerative illness still abounds. In addition to Candida, incidence of heart and blood vessel disease, hypertension, arteriosclerosis, cancer, diabetes, arthritis, obesity, neuro-muscular illness, and other degenerative diseases continue to increase.

However, some progress has been made! Due to the promotion of nutrition by a few enlightened doctors, many nutritionists, and other health food advocates, organizations such as the American Heart Association and the National Cancer Institute have finally jumped on the nutrition band wagon. In one advertisement by the American Cancer Society, next to a picture of a grocer holding an armload of vegetables, the copy reads, "He may not look like everybody's idea of a cancer specialist. But there's strong evidence that your greengrocer has access to cancer protection you won't find in any doctor's office." The ad concludes with the appeal, "In short, make sure you do what your mother always told you to do. Eat your vegetables."

Advertisements such as this are the result of a study conducted in the early '80s by the National Cancer Institute. NCI spent over two million dollars coming to a very startling conclusion: lifestyles, such as diet, are a factor in 9 out of 10 cases of cancer. And to follow that simple logic, one might conclude that by changing lifestyles, one could greatly reduce the likelihood of getting cancer — by as much as the same 90 percent. One study at Harvard University showed that the chances of dying from cancer can be reduced by 70 percent if two or more portions of vegetables and fruit are consumed everyday. They also recommended a reduction of fat and cholesterol, as well as other lifestyle changes. Similar links can be found to coronary heart disease and other chronic illnesses.

So, these studies confirm the fact that a nutritious diet does definitely correlate with prevention of illness. It's encouraging to see more of an emphasis on nutrition by these organizations that have traditionally been more involved in the treatment of, rather than the prevention of, disease. But they have only uncovered the tip of the iceberg. While these changes are all desirable, even more improvements in diet are necessary in order to obtain optimum health.

Making poor food choices is often due to a lack of proper nutrition education as well as to being unaware of certain food processing techniques that create nutritionally "dead" food. How can dead food keep people alive? The previous chapter focused on improving the digestive system through regulation. It is also vital to improve the digestive system by carefully considering food choices.

Are All Food Groups Good For Us?

Since early childhood, we have traditionally been taught to eat from the basic food groups: grains, vegetables/fruits, meat, and dairy. Aside from social conditioning of families and peers, major advertising campaigns have also attempted to convince people that they must partake of all four food groups, especially meat and milk, in order to remain healthy. But are all of these foods really healthy? In examining the meat, eggs, and dairy food groups below, one may be surprised to learn that these foods are not so "ideal" and actually do more to **delay** digestion than any other food group.

Meat

Even though meat consumption has steadily increased over the last several decades, organizations such as the American Heart Association and the American Cancer Society are now advising a reduction of meat intake. Obviously, health experts are catching on to the correlation between disease and meat consumption. Could it be possible that humans were not meant to eat meat? Many people find it surprising that there are numerous physiological differences between humans and the animals that were designed to eat meat. For example:

—Humans belong to a category of mammals who are plant eaters, called herbivores. They must chew their food in order to digest it, as opposed to a carnivorous animal (meat eater) that can swallow its food whole. Human teeth have sharp cutting incisors used for biting off pieces of food and flat nodular molars used for crushing and grinding food. These teeth were designed to break down fruits, vegetables, seeds, and nuts. On the other hand, carnivorous animals with elongated, sharp-pointed teeth grasp and tear their food, such as raw meat, with little chewing.

—Human hands also offer proof of being predisposed herbivores; they are designed for gathering, not tearing or ripping flesh as a carnivore's are.

—Humans have an enzyme in their saliva called alpha-amylase, which is necessary to break down complex carbohydrates found in plant foods, in their saliva. Carnivores do not produce this enzyme.

—Humans drink water by sipping, while carnivores lap it up. Humans cool their bodies by perspiring, while carnivores pant.

In addition to the above, there is another very important physiological difference between herbivores and carnivores: the digestive tract. A carnivore has a very short digestive tract (transit time is approximately 6 hours or less) so that when it consumes flesh, it is broken down very quickly. In this way, the carnivore voids itself of harmful residues and the likelihood of putrefaction or other damage to the digestive system. And even though animals eat flesh food that is low in fiber and high in cholesterol, fat, and protein, they have the necessary components in their digestive tract to break down these harmful elements.

On the other hand, a human's intestines are much longer, allowing ample time to digest complex carbohydrates from high-fiber foods such as fruits, vegetables, seeds, and nuts. As opposed to the six-hour transit time (the time it takes for food to make its way through the body) for carnivores, the transit time provided by the human digestive tract is 24-30 hours.

When humans eat meat this ideal transit time is greatly affected for two reasons: First, their systems cannot efficiently break down the excessive fat, protein, and cholesterol. Second, the lack of fiber in meat slows its descent through the intestines, causing it to remain in the system for approximately *88 hours!!! That's right, it takes an average of 88 hours for meat to make its way through the digestive system as opposed to the 24 to 30 hours it would take for the diet humans were designed to eat!*

Now, pay close attention to this: If meat is allowed to remain in human intestines for approximately 88 hours at about 98 degrees in a dark, damp climate, what will occur? *Fermentation.* Fermentation in the intestine is equally as harmful as that in the stomach. First of all, as discussed in the previous chapter, this fermentation encourages a perfect environment in which microorganisms, including yeast, can thrive. Second, a putrefying process takes place that allows the high protein content of meat to create chemicals that are dangerous and many times carcinogenic (cancer-causing) to the entire body. In future chapters, alarming facts will be revealed concerning how chemicals currently being added to meat are increasing an already severe health problem.

Besides being low in fiber, meat contains high amounts of fat, cholesterol, and protein that other human organs struggle to break down. What happens to the excess? It is absorbed in the tissues of the body, potentially to resurface later in the form of clogged arteries, heart disease, and other illnesses. However, if the diet is composed of healthy foods from the bean (legume), whole grain, vegetable, fruit, nut, and seed families, transit time is normal (providing all digestion principles are followed and fermentation does not occur). Hence, yeast growth is not encouraged.

For those afraid of missing the flavor of meat, perhaps knowing what gives meat its flavor will make its absence a little fonder. Fat, blood, and uric acid all contribute to the flavor of a piece of meat, especially red meat. Subsequently, people who eat meat have a higher amount of uric acid in *their* urine, proof that an animal's waste products contained in meat transfer into the human body despite cooking procedures.

A common misconception is that anything harmful in meat will be destroyed during the cooking process. Wrong! Just as pasteurization does not guarantee the safety of milk, cooking does not destroy all contaminants in meats. True, some types of bacteria can be destroyed by cooking; however, viruses are more stubborn. For example, foot and mouth disease viruses can survive 176 degrees Fahrenheit cooking temperatures. Well-done roast beef may only reach about 168.8 degrees Fahrenheit with rare roast beef reaching only 140 degrees Fahrenheit. Many organisms, including bacteria and viruses, can survive normal cooking temperatures. It would be necessary to cook meat at higher temperatures and for longer periods of time than is normally done in every home and restaurant in order to totally eliminate most exposure to disease.

Many animals suffer from disease, just as humans do, be it cancer, hepatitis, herpes, leukemia, arthritis, or many others also. Unfortunately, a diet including meat will most likely include these diseases. It may be difficult to believe that all animals are not tested for contamination before and during the slaughtering process. Yes, there are certain guidelines, but these are vague and not always followed. Meat inspectors are given too much to inspect in too little time. For example, a meat inspector is given an average of *eight seconds* to examine a 1500-pound steer to determine if it is fit for human consumption. Comparably, it requires two and one-half hours for a pathologist to examine the body of a 150-pound man. Even if the inspector did find a questionable situation, samples of the carcass are not taken and sent to a laboratory for analysis. Instead, reports abound of meat-packing plants slicing off visible tumors from an animal, then continuing to process the rest of the carcass for human consumption. Since cancer in animals is nearly always a virus and more than likely has spread to all other tissues of the body, cutting off the tumor does not limit the consumer's exposure to the cancer virus.

And what about animals who are diseased but show no signs of it? As shown by these instances, a consumer is never aware of eating diseased meat. In 1987, a Food Safety and Inspection Service official, Vernie Gee, testified before a Senate subcommittee that the government label normally stamped on beef, poultry, and pork, "USDA Inspected and Approved," should be changed to "Eat At Your Own Risk." Because of mismanagement, poor training, and the almighty dollar, contaminated meat is making its way to the dinner table *every* day.

Fish

Many people have been eating fish for years and boasting of its healthful properties. Years ago that fact was more true. But that was before man started to contaminate the waters. There have been incidents where several waste disposal companies illegally dumped hospital waste into certain waters in this country. Reports indicated that among those substances were human parts, blood samples (including some contaminated with the AIDS virus), and other infectious wastes. Into New England coastal waters have been dumped more than one trillion gallons of sewage, industrial wastewater, and polluted storm water, according to a researcher affiliated with an environmental group called the Coast Alliance. Fish from today's contaminated waters can actually transport to humans many viruses such as coxsackie, rheo, and polio viruses.

Undercooked fish has long been a source of parasite and worm infestation in man. However, the Center for Disease Control in Atlanta reports a tremendous increase in known cases of tapeworm due to the increasing popularity of eating raw fish such as sushi. But for every known case, there are many that remain unknown. Victims could be suffering from symptoms such as numb sensations in the extremities, fatigue, weakness, weight gain or loss, malabsorption of food, and many others.

Eggs

Unfortunately, eggs are responsible for a large portion of chronic illnesses today, especially allergies. For example, egg white contains histamine-like products that can produce various allergic reactions. Other common symptoms are urethritis, cystitis, gastrointestinal problems, skin disorders, and conjunctival infections. Virtually every single egg harbors bacteria that are not always killed by cooking processes. A temperature of at least *350 degrees for 30 minutes is necessary in order to kill bacteria.*Many cooking methods, including baking, frying, and boiling, do not attain either adequate temperature, length of time, or both. Naturally, any product that contains either raw eggs (such as ice cream, protein drinks or dried egg products) or eggs cooked for less than the recommended time is a source of infection.

Milk and Milk Products

Cows' milk is a product that has been touted as the "perfect food" for adults as well as children. Yet doesn't it seem strange that, of all mammals, humans are the only ones that continue to drink milk after early childhood? Even if someone wanted to continue drinking milk, wouldn't it make more sense to drink milk from their own species rather than that of another? Or, if milk is so important for growth, why not drink dog milk, or even rat milk? Due to the extremely high fat and protein composition of these milks, their offspring are able to double their birth weight in just days, while humans take months.

The "perfectness" of milk, promoted by milk producers, should be called the "milk myth." Even though their claims that milk is a nutrient-rich food are true, these nutrients are not ideal for humans. Just like meat, milk is a concentrated product that is hard to break down. It is high in fat, protein, and salt, but low in Vitamin C, zinc, and iron. This combination of nutrients is perfectly suited for baby cows, allowing them to double their birth weight in only 47 days and reach an ultimate weight of approximately 300 pounds in 12 months! Also, cows have four stomachs in which to "process" this nutrient-rich food. Humans only have one stomach and cannot properly assimilate the complex structure of components such as milk sugars, milk protein, and butter fat. Therefore, these components end up doing more damage to the body than good, often resulting in allergies. Milk allergies are sometimes a mystery since the symptoms do not always appear at the time the product is consumed. Bloating, dizziness, colitis, bodyaches, and headaches are just a few of the numerous symptoms milk intolerance can produce.

Another very serious health hazard of milk is the fact that it is only pasteurized, not sterilized. And there is a difference! Pasteurization temperatures are not high enough to kill certain bacteria and many viruses, such as the Rauscher/Moloney murine leukemia viruses and the Moloney and Rous sarcoma viruses (which are cancer-producing viruses). As a result, childhood leukemia is much higher among children who consume milk.

Cheese

It seems that everybody loves cheese. Just as with meat, cheese is believed to be a beneficial food necessary to good health. Even those who have decided to leave meat out of their diet, lacto-ovo vegetarians, usually rely heavily on cheese products for their protein intake. However, cheese lovers may be surprised to learn exactly what happens in the cheese-making process. For instance, many are not aware that:

—Most milk used to make cheese is not even pasteurized, let alone sterilized. Therefore, eating cheese carries more threat of bacteria and viruses than does drinking milk. Several imported cheeses were found to have as many as 600 germs in a teaspoon!

—Cheese is created from the waste products of unpasteurized milk. It is fermented, which produces mold, bacteria, toxic alkaloids, and amines, which have been shown to cause seizures, headaches (including migraine), high blood pressure, palpitations, allergies, and more. Additionally, the fermentation process also produces irritating fatty and lactic acids, ammonia, and other chemicals, some of which are carcinogenic.

—In order to curdle the milk in cheese, rennet is used. It is usually derived from calves' stomachs and is used in combination with an enzyme, normally from a hog's stomach. Most vegetarians are not aware that actual parts of a cow or hog are normally used in making cheese.

When considering the health benefits of cheese, look over the descriptive words that describe the cheese-making process: bacteria, virus, waste products, fermentation, toxic, irritating, carcinogenic, calves' stomach, mold, hog's stomach, etc. The bottom line is that any product that is a result of a reaction to bacteria and fermentation cannot be healthy. Actually, cheese does not have an appealing taste except that people have been conditioned to like it. The fact is, it tastes spoiled because it is spoiled! However, people learn from an early age to acquire a taste for it because they are told over and over how good it tastes and how good it is for them!

An important point to remember is that any by-product from an animal, including eggs, cheese, yogurt, milk (evaporated, non-fat and dry), and ice cream, has the potential to transmit disease, just as meat does. After all, these are all by-products of animals. Whatever disease or condition from which an animal is suffering will also be present in its by-products. Also, the high protein content of these foods not only adds unnecessary calories to the diet, but is taxing to all digestive organs, contributing to various types of degenerative disease. Any so-called nutritional benefits from animal products or by-products can be obtained quite adequately through the use of other wholesome foods, which will be discussed in Chapter 5.

Below are some of the more common diseases that can actually be transmitted from animal foods to humans:

CHICKEN/EGGS/TURKEY

Leucosis (leukemia)	Salmonellosis
Newcastle Disease	Histoplasmosis Malignant Lymphoma

BEEF/MILK/CHEESE

Salmonellosis	Staphylococci
Ringworm	Tetanus
Herpes	Parasites
Rabies	Actinomycosis
Scarlet Fever	Diptheria
Polio	Brucellosis
Streptococci	Foot & Mouth Disease

PORK

Trichinosis	Meningitis
Sporotrotrichosis	Staphylococci
Brucellosis	

FISH/SEAFOOD

Polio Virus	Coxsackie Virus
Rheo Virus	Tapeworms
Hepatitis	

Contact With Live Animals and Pets

It is important to be aware that live animals and pets can also pose a health threat to humans. Most house pets are fed pet food, which is even more inferior than human food. It poses a higher contamination risk because there are fewer processing guidelines. Waste animal parts that are rancid and bacteria-laden are often used, transmitting viruses, worms, and parasites to animals. This food is also high in protein and low in complex carbohydrates, providing a perfect pH balance for bacteria and disease. Naturally, this often results in more illness and shortened life spans for animals.

Animals who venture outside, even for short periods of time, are exposed to fleas, mosquitos, ticks, and flies, creatures that often carry germs or organisms of serious diseases, such as Lyme disease or Rocky

Mountain spotted fever. Although humans can also be directly infected by these insects, chances are not as great. Animals can actually carry worm and parasite larvae or bacteria on their bodies, especially their paws, as they go in and out of the home. Depending on the strength of the animals' immune systems, they will either resist or fall prey to some of these illnesses. Naturally, if they resist, their owners will never know they were infected. However, they are still a carrier of disease to humans. Even though the animals do not show signs of infection, they can still be infected, exposing humans as well.

For example, authorities on pet/animal transmitted diseases cite cats, more than other pets, as prominent carriers of disease. Fleas, bites, or scratches from cats transmit many diseases, including toxoplasmosis. Often mistaken for flu in adults, this disease can actually cause blindness or premature death in the children of mothers who where infected during pregnancy. It can also result in other serious disorders that may not become apparent until early adulthood, such as mental retardation, deformities, eye problems, and other neurological disease. (A person can also be exposed to toxoplasmosis from eating raw or undercooked meat and from contact with various livestock and pets other than cats.)

It is virtually impossible to keep an animal as clean as a human. Humans bathe daily, animals do not. Therefore, they carry bacteria on their bodies, which encourages fleas and other critters to harbor there. Also, the feces of animals may contain bacteria, worms, parasites, and other microorganisms. Unlike humans, pets do not use toilet paper; therefore, when they come back into the house, contamination is often transferred to furniture, floors, beds, clothing, and humans. Many times, people will sit down to eat right after handling a pet that has just defecated, not realizing the possibility of disease transmission. Yet most people laugh at the thought of contracting diseases such as worms or parasites from their pets!

Below are some of the more common diseases that can be transmitted from live animals to humans:

PETS

Leptospirosis	Ringworm
Hookworm	Roundworm
Lice	Mites
Erysipelas	Brucellosis
Papular Urticaria	Salmonella
Rabies	Toxoplasmosis
Pasteurella Multocida	Psittacosis
Lymphocytic Choriomeningitis	Herpes Virus
Measles	Encephalitis
Hepatitis	Tuberculosis
Giardia lamblia	

Another source of exposure to worms, parasites, and bacteria is working or playing outside. Although rare for adults, children often contact bacteria in this way. Worms and parasites often lay their eggs in the grass, sand, and/or dirt. These eggs are too small to be detected by the human eye but fit perfectly under the fingernail of a small child. Although less of a threat, there are even bacteria-laden spores in the air that can be inhaled. Likewise, walking barefoot in the grass or dirt can be an open invitation to unwanted creatures. In rare instances, hookworms have been known to burrow themselves into human skin, usually through the soles of the feet.

It is still possible to enjoy pets and the great outdoors by following a few guidelines that will reduce exposure to microorganistic infestation, such as:

Diet—By eliminating the consumption of meat and dairy products, a large risk of disease will be eliminated. A wholesome diet can create a pH balance that will not support infestations. In fact, some people say they notice indications of worm infestations being eliminated in their feces, usually in the first few months of the 3-C Program. Be assured that as dietary improvements strengthen the immune system, all microorganisms will be reduced. After several months on this program, if a stubborn case of infestation remains, there are several herbal preparations that can help. If an herbal treatment is implemented, keep in mind that herbs should always be used with caution. Consult a master herbalist, keep the treatment program simple by using a preparation of only one or two herbs, and use it only long enough to accomplish the goal. Then, if necessary, the treatment can be repeated at a later time. (See Chapter 5, Internal Cleansers.)

Pets—Because pets are a definite risk of transmitting disease, they should, preferably, be kept outside. Sharing a home with pets is inviting trouble. At the very least, all pets should receive a daily dose of either raw garlic or a good garlic supplement to help fight viral, bacterial, and parasitic infestations. Do not kiss pets, sleep with them, or handle their feces. Always, ALWAYS wash hands thoroughly after handling animals. Try to limit walking barefoot in the grass or dirt and keep in mind that anything that lives outside can harbor disease. Flies, fleas, ticks, and other insects may infect pets and animals; they, in turn, can infect people.

Symptoms of Animal-Transmitted Diseases

When the body is first exposed to microorganistic infestations, such as worms or parasites, the original symptoms usually mock food poisoning or flu virus to varying degrees, depending on the amount transmitted and the condition of the immune system. Common symptoms can include: fever, muscle aches, chills, abdominal pain, swelling, weakness, dizziness, rashes, and diarrhea. Other symptoms can include numbness of the extremities, meningitis, kidney problems, and blood poisoning.

Even though the initial symptoms usually pass, not all organisms leave the body. Trichina, for instance, can settle in the large muscles of the body, and as a natural body defense the immune system produces antibodies in an attempt to fight this infestation. This defense action of the immune system allows the body to cope with the invader, producing a "false" recovery. But the battle has only begun, because parasitic organisms often behave like animals living in the human body. (An interesting fact is that parasitic organisms include all types of worms, protozoa, mold, and fungus, including Candida.) They complete life cycles similar to other animals in that they eat, excrete their wastes, and reproduce. Some types can survive on any diet, but most prefer a pH level resulting from junk food diets high in sugar and processed foods and low in whole foods. After robbing a person of nourishment, they dump their toxic wastes into that person's system. It's like having a small dose of poison every day, resulting in a wide range of symptoms, such as anemia, allergies, constipation, diarrhea, indigestion, acne, eczema, seborrhea and other skin disorders, bloating, weight gain or loss, and many other non-specific complaints.

Coping with the toxic overload produced by these microorganisms weakens the immune system. Add to this poor lifestyle choices such as improper diet, stress, and lack of exercise, and it's no wonder that illness is the result.

When will it be possible to pinpoint exactly the number of diseases transmitted to man from animals? Until this area of study is brought to the attention of more researchers, it will remain uncertain. However, there is enough data available now to encourage people to view exposure of microorganisms as a very real threat of illness. Sadly, most physicians do not even realize a possible connection between illness and microorganistic infestation. Many times this is due to the fact that initial encounters with microorganisms may be short-term, often mimicking flu symptoms. Although initial symptoms usually subside, the possibility of these organisms producing subsequent illness is very real. Naturally, due to varying lifestyle choices and habits, not all people are exposed to the same organisms.

There are some experts who believe that types of microorganistic or communicable diseases can suppress the immune system to the point of causing death, even though the cause of death is usually not listed as communicable disease. In order to verify that fact, it would take a highly-trained pathologist several hours in autopsy time and several weeks of study under a microscope performing chemical and bacterial testing. It simply isn't feasible, time-wise or dollar-wise. The bottom line is: Even though doctors don't talk about microorganistic diseases and most people aren't aware of them, they remain a very real threat to society.

Chemicals—Invisible Ingredients In Food

It is amazing to learn how food has become so adulterated in today's world. Presenting all pertinent information regarding the use of food-related chemicals and how they affect human health would be impossible in this limited space. However, there are many good books that deal with this subject in great depth.

Chemicals appear in almost every commercially prepared food. The problem is that most people have either been sold a bill of goods regarding the safety of certain chemicals or they may be totally unaware of their existence because they do not appear on the label. Government agencies such as the Department of Agriculture and Commerce, the Food and Drug Administration, and the Federal Trade Commission have developed certain guidelines regulating the use of chemicals in food for public sale. Included in these guidelines are types of chemicals that can be used, what quantities can be used, and whether or not they must appear on the label, which can be misleading to the consumer. For instance:

Labeling

—A food label is not required to reveal certain ingredients in a product, such as additives, flavorings, spices, fats, colorings, and sulfites.

—If a chemical, such as a preservative, is added to an ingredient before that ingredient is processed into the final food product, not only does the preservative not have to appear on the ingredient label, but the label can actually claim "no preservatives." But it's still in there.

—Numerous manufacturing contaminants accidentally find their way into food during the shipping, storage, and production phases. Chemicals such as oils, solvents, detergents, plastics, and lubricating oils do not have to appear on ingredient labels simply because they were not intended to be an ingredient.

—Many foods contain chemicals that are not listed on the label because those chemicals are used in quantities at or below a specified amount regulated by the government. For instance, products labeled "no artificial flavors" or "no preservatives" may actually contain them.

—Because there exists no FDA definition as to what is "natural" or "organic," a manufacturer can falsely label any product in this manner.

Additive Usage

—Government guidelines dictate what chemicals and how much of them can be added to food. However, what might be safe for one person may not be safe for another. Sulfites, a preservative, will not kill everyone who eats them, but they have been responsible for the deaths of at least a small number of people. In addition, all that is necessary in order for the FDA to permit additive usage is for the manufacturer to declare that a product is safe, even though that declaration is based on very limited testing. To add insult to injury, testing on certain additives is not usually completed by an independent laboratory but by the manufacturer themselves! Naturally, their test results are going to promote the safety of their product, as well as their profits. Some examples of additives and their sources would be nitrates and nitrites in bacon, BHT and BHA in breakfast cereals, and MSG in barbecue potato chips.

—Some additives posing tremendous health threats are pesticides, insecticides, antibiotics, and hormones. Between two and three billion pounds of dangerous pesticides used by this country's farmers end up in food every year.

There are more than 550 insecticides used in this country today, of which only a small number have been tested for safety — mostly on animals. Over 478 million dollars worth of antibiotics (55 percent of all antibiotics produced in the U.S.) are added to animal feed every year. These antibiotics accumulate in the flesh of animals, which is then sold to the public for consumption. Consequently, consumers of meat, eggs and dairy products are also ingesting antibiotics without realizing it. Aside from the fact that antibiotics reduce the good bacteria in the body, consuming them regularly (even "second-hand" through animal products) will cause the body to develop an immunity to these antibiotics. Should the need for antibiotics arise in an emergency situation, they could be ineffective.

Hormones have an entirely different affect on animals and people than antibiotics. Thyroid hormones (growth hormones) are given to cows to increase their milk yields, or to "fatten" them up in half the normal time. Since it has been established that these hormones do pass through the cow and into its milk, it is safe to assume that people who are drinking milk are also being affected by these growth hormones. If these hormones can increase a cow's growth potential in less time, is it no wonder children today look and act like they are 18 years old when they are actually 13 years old? Suffice it to say that the composite effect of years of adding antibiotics and growth hormones to food sources has yet to rear its ugly head.

At this point, a close examination of the limitations of the Federal Government as a food additive regulator is in order. Isn't it ironic that government regulations claim that an additive is not harmful unless it is consumed in large quantities? When considering the number of foods in today's supermarkets that contain additives, they ARE being consumed in large quantities. It is the sum total of all these additives that contribute to health problems.

Chemicals in food, water, and medications definitely weaken the immune system, thereby adding to the list of elements that can increase the risk of Candida and other illnesses. Many times, Candida patients will make improvements simply by limiting their chemical exposure. That's why, in the 3-C Program, it is so necessary to be very particular about the quality of food, water, and anything else put into the body. However, even after a recovery from Candida, one should still be acutely aware of how damaging chemicals can be, even to healthy individuals.

WATER/3-C PRINCIPLE

Water is even more important to life than food. Many people don't realize that the cells of the body are comprised of 60 to 90 percent water. Think of it! In all the components of the human body — muscles, bones, skin, organs — water is the most prevalent element, yet the most neglected. Water saturates the tissues in the body to keep them in proper working order, helps to replenish the supply of saliva, transports nutrients from food into cells, regulates body temperature, and keeps the kidneys, which are the waterworks factory of the body, running smoothly. Each day the kidneys filter about fifty gallons of liquid to aid the digestive tract, which needs water to produce approximately eight quarts of digestive juice. Two to four quarts of water are lost every day through the skin, lungs, intestinal tract, and kidneys. In addition, chemicals contained in caffeinated products and cigarettes act as diuretics, causing further water loss. Since the body cannot produce water on its own, it is vital that enough be consumed to replenish what is lost.

All water is not the same. While everyone needs good quality water, this is especially important for those working to regain good health. Can it be found at every kitchen sink? Consider several chemicals commonly added to water:

Flouride (also found in toothpaste)—Flourides attack almost everything. According to Dr. H.W. Holderby in his *Report On Water,* "The chemical action of flourides is such that all containers must be lined with rubber or plastic, for it eats through all metal material. What must it do to the tissues of the body? It can also unite with other chemicals, forming further dangerous compounds...medical authorities now state it can cause cancer, Mongoloid births, kidney disorders, bone diseases, impotency and even madness." Other studies have shown that fluoride interferes with the proper growth of children and the essential repair and function of many parts of the body.

The recommended daily requirement of fluoride necessary to prevent tooth decay is one milligram, which is obtained from four glasses of water at the average rate of 1 part per milligram. However, concentrations of 1.5 parts per milligram are reported in many water systems, and most people drink more than four glasses of water per day, whether from the faucet or in juices, soda pop, alcoholic beverages, food, and so on. At this rate, "normal" daily consumption has been labeled as toxic, even by the United States Public Health Service.

Chlorine—While chlorine does kill bacteria, this action creates decomposing organic material in the water supply, which leads to the formation of cancer-causing compounds called trihalomethanes. Dr. Richard Harris says, "The practice of chlorinating public drinking water appears to increase the risk of gastrointestinal cancer over a person's lifetime by between 50 and

100 percent." Even though chlorine is supposed to eradicate viruses, bacteria, and parasites, it is not totally successful. The Center for Disease Control in Atlanta says the number of reported cases of giardiasis (a parasite) increases by thousands every year. Outbreaks have been reported in many major cities. In spite of this, physicians are not required to report giardiasis to public health officials! Obviously, chlorine is not the answer to all microorganistic infestations.

Pesticides, Herbicides and Other Chemicals—According to *The State of the Environment*, a report published in 1985 by the Organization for Economic Co-operation and Development, groundwater in many areas is contaminated by nitrates and pesticides used in intensive agriculture, by urban run-off, and by seepage from abandoned contaminated sites. Soil is being treated today with more and more chemicals as herbicides are used to replace weeding. The report stated, "More sophisticated methods of measurement and analysis have led to a gradual identification of a wider range of pollutants in air, water and soil, including organic substances such as PCB's and chlorofluorocarbons; metals such as lead, cadmium and mercury; and a number of fibers such as asbestos and fiberglass." All of these new pollutants supposedly reflect "progress" in the modern way of life. However, it may be more realistic to say that people are quickly being wisked away toward the 21st century on a toxic cloud!

Gene Rosov is president of WaterTest Corporation, the nations's largest independent drinking-water testing laboratory. In testifying before Congress on water quality, Mr. Rosov said that poor-quality water is not only a result of chemicals added to water at treatment plants but also of the contamination that occurs after the water leaves the plant. Metal contaminants from pipes, as well as back-flow into the water line from air conditioners, stopped-up toilets and sinks, and other sources all contribute to poor water. Unfortunately, these go undetected since utilities are only required to test the water they provide to consumers from the point of origin. Obviously, a lot can happen between there and the kitchen faucet!

Actually, there are many different kinds of water: rain, snow, hard, soft, raw, tap, boiled, filtered, de-ionized, reverse osmosis, and distilled. A brief discussion of each one follows:

—Rain water and snow water have been "distilled" by the heat of the sun and should contain no mineral matter or germs; however by the time these waters fall through the polluted air, they are full of all types of bacteria.

—Hard water and soft water are waters that have run through or over the ground in any way, and they comprise most of the available drinking water. They contain, in various degrees, all types of minerals, nitrates, chlorides, viruses, bacteria, and many other harmful minerals and chemicals. So-called "mineral waters" from springs are supposed to have beneficial effects. However, according to Dr. Allen Banik, "The reason mineral waters have this so-called medicinal effect is because the body tries to throw off excess minerals which invade it as intruding foreign deposits." In fact, some researchers feel that certain minerals may team up with cholesterol to create the plaque that causes arteriosclerosis.

Soft water has been artificially softened through the use of excess amounts of salt; some people may consider water to be naturally soft if it came from rivers and lakes. Either way, considering the amount of pollution in waters today, it is no wonder Jacques Cousteau was quoted as saying, "Each year the earth's rivers carry to sea five billion tons of dissolved minerals and other unnumbered millions of tons of carbon compounds and factory pollutants. Ocean life has decreased 40 percent the last 20 years."

—Raw or "tap" water can be either hard or soft but has not been boiled. It contains viruses, bacteria, and chemicals. As discussed above, even though chlorination treatments kill some germs and viruses, they also destroy healthy cells. Unfortunately, it has been reported that much of the "bottled" water purchased in this country is nothing more than tap water. Therefore, most bottled water still carries all the risks of tap water.

—Boiled water is advantageous only due to the fact that boiling destroys most bacteria. However, drinking "dead germs" creates bacterial food that encourages the growth of unfriendly "live" bacteria in the body.

—Filtered water has typically been thought to be purified. Even though some calcium and other solid substances are removed through filtering, filters do not adequately trap all viruses and bacteria. In addition, the bacteria that filters do trap provide an excellent breeding ground for additional bacteria. As a result, the filter eventually contains more germs than the water poured through it.

—De-ionized water has had minerals removed and is probably the next best to distilled. However, resin beds used in this process provide a perfect breeding ground for bacteria.

— Reverse osmosis water is purified by forcing a portion of water through a membrane. Substantial amounts of contaminants are removed during this process, but the degree of purity can vary widely depending on types and conditions of equipment used. Also, the membrane will eventually conatin more germs than the water that passes through it.

—Distilled water is the purest form available. Distilled water has been vaporized, and the rising vapors cannot hold anything, including viruses, bacteria, waste products, or other harmful substances. All contaminants are left behind. This vapor condenses into pure water. Because of the increased amounts of chemicals, such as chlorine and fluoride, that cities are putting into water supplies, it may be necessary to also post-filter distilled water in order to remove these additional chemicals.

A common assumption is that distilled water may leach minerals out of the body. Keep in mind that leaching cannot occur once the mineral becomes part of a cell system. Distilled water only leaches excess or harmful minerals from the body. In addition to this, the body cannot assimilate inorganic minerals, which most waters contain. Plants have the ability to convert inorganic minerals into organic minerals, which people can then eat and utilize. Consuming hard water full of inorganic minerals which the body cannot break down, much like concentrated food, produces many adverse effects such as arthritis, constipation, hardened arteries, and kidney or liver stones.

Distilled water can also help to excrete excessive heavy metals from the body. Much disease and sickness today is compounded by an accumulation of metals such as arsenic, aluminum, asbestos, iron, cadmium, copper, mercury, and lead. All of these contaminants contribute to a toxic overload that weakens the immune system, leaving the body unprotected from various illness.

For all of these reasons, it is imperative that only distilled water be consumed while utilizing the 3-C Program. The main objective is to eliminate exposure to microorganisms while reducing accumulated deposits of harmful minerals and heavy metals. If would be difficult to become mineral-deficient if properly following the 3-C Diet. Likewise, supplementing with a mineral compound is not necessary as long as a proper diet is maintained. Supplements are expensive, concentrated, and often not well-absorbed.

Water Requirements For The 3-C Program

An easy method to determine how many ounces of water the body requires every day is to divide body weight in half. Then, divide this figure by 8 in order to determine how many 8-ounce glasses it would take to fulfill that requirement. For instance, a 100-pound person would require 50 ounces of water everyday. Divide those ounces by 8, and that comes out to a little over six glasses of water per day to fulfill that person's water requirement. If water is lost through perspiration for any reason such as exercise, hot weather, strenuous work, or fever, water requirements should be increased. Another easy method to determine if enough water is being consumed is to check the color of the urine; it should be almost colorless. If it is not, drink more water.

Due to the *Kyolic* liquid garlic and dietary changes, the body will be cleansing many toxins at the beginning of the 3-C Program. While this is desirable, a little more than the normal requirement of water is necessary to aid the body in this process. Therefore, the daily minimum water requirement should be increased by 50 percent. For example, if a person weighs 128 pounds, normally 64 ounces of water per day would be required (8 glasses). But, when initiating the 3-C Program, that same 128-pound person would require an additional 50 percent, or 4 extra glasses, totaling 12 glasses of water per day.

Once the proper daily amount of water consumption has been determined, the guidelines below will help in knowing when to consume water:

— Water should *always* be consumed *between meals* but *never with* meals.

— Water intake should be discontinued 30 minutes before each meal and not resumed until 60 minutes after each meal. Waiting up to 90 minutes after a meal to drink water is even better.

— Most of the daily water requirement should be consumed by late afternoon so that sleep is not interrupted at night with frequent trips to the bathroom. A handy way to keep track of water intake is to fill a gallon jug with one's daily requirement first thing in the morning. After drinking the first two glasses out of this, the balance should be divided between morning and late afternoon (of course, between meals), saving only one glass for evening.

— It is best to drink water at room temperature. Ingesting any food or liquid too hot or too cold can **delay** the absorption and digestion process.

The Use Of Herbal Teas

Herbal teas make a wonderful substitute for more harmful drinks such as coffee, caffeinated tea, soft drinks, or alcohol. One herbal tea, Pau d' Arco, has been used in treating Candida, due to its antifungal properties. However, the use of herbal teas is not recommended while completing the Getting Well segment of the 3-C Program for several reasons. First of all, experience has shown that the use of the 3-C principles can assist in reduction of yeast without the use of herbal teas. Second, it is easy to forget that herbal teas are made from herbs, which can have strong medicinal properties, some of which may cause an increase in the cleansing or die-off reaction that would not be pleasant. Third, even though they are liquid products, herbal teas do require a degree of digestion.

Different people may react differently to herbal teas. For some, certain herbal teas act as diuretics, upsetting the kidneys. Drinking some herbal teas (licorice tea, for example) in large quantities could cause high blood pressure, retention of sodium, loss of potassium, and diarrhea. Some people have even reported gastrointestinal problems from drinking chamomile tea, which is normally quite safe and is even promoted for soothing the stomach. Keep in mind that someone with an allergy to ragweed, asters, or chrysanthemums might also adversely react to teas containing flowers of golden rod, marigold, or yarrow. Also, be careful when mixing herbs or herbal teas. Two seemingly-innocent herbs may become quite potent when combined.

This is not to say that herbs are always harmful. Conversely, they are marvelous medicine for short-term, therapeutic use, as well as for an enjoyable beverage. (See Chapter 5, Internal Cleansers.) However, using large amounts of them with no herbal knowledge is especially unwise for Candida patients who tend to be over-sensitive. Many times it is easy to overdo with herbs when using them as teas because the connection is not made between a simple beverage and a medicinal effect.

When one has reached Staying Well there are several mild herbal teas that may be included in the diet. Little known danger has been reported with teas such as alfalfa, barley, chicory, red clover, hops (not wild hops, which is toxic), rose hips, lemongrass, or mint. If they are consumed weak and in no more than a two-herb combination, they are normally very safe.

Fruit Juices

Even if fruit was permitted in the Getting Well segment, fruit juice would not be recommended for Candida patients for several reasons. First of all, commercial fruit juices are very likely to be fermented from lengthy processing times, which may account for setbacks in the progress of Candida patients who have been drinking fruit juice. Second, even healthy people need to know that drinking any fruit juice, even freshly made, causes the digestive process to start over again. Obviously, this causes **delay** in the digestion of the previous meal, which causes fermentation. Third, fruit juice is a concentrated product, as discussed in Chapter 3. In this form it acts more as a simple sugar, as opposed to a complex sugar, and enters the bloodstream very quickly. Fruit should be eaten in its whole state because then the fiber and pulp of the fruit slow down the sugar-releasing process.

Water Cleanses Outside As Well As Inside

Many toxins are eliminated through the skin, which is the largest eliminative organ of the body. Every day, this occurs naturally, increasing during times of heavy perspiration, as in hot weather or during exercise. Many Candida patients do not perspire in the beginning of the program. However, perspiration should be viewed as an important aid to recovery and also as a sign that the adrenal glands are working more efficiently. The main goal here is to help the body eliminate toxins in as many ways as possible: through a good diet, exercise, additional water intake, perspiration, *Kyolic* liquid garlic, and so forth.

The skin is not only capable of elimination but of absorption, as well. As perspiration eliminates toxins through the pores, the skin can also reabsorb them. For this reason it is important to shower every day, especially immediately after exercise. An additional shower can be taken in the evening, particularly during the first few weeks of the 3-C Program as toxin elimination is greater. Use a loofah sponge (a natural fiber sponge available at most health food stores) or brush to help remove accumulated impurities on the skin's outer surface. They can be periodically boiled to keep free of bacteria. A natural glycerine soap is preferred to the common bath bar that may contain chemicals. Keeping the skin and clothes clean will ensure that toxins are not reabsorbed by the skin.

Water is such an important element that although a person can survive without food for many days, one can only go a few days without water. The use of water sustains and cleanses the body and is a valuable treatment (hydrotherapy) for many illnesses such as sinus headaches, viruses, infections, and much, much more. *Hydrotherapy* and *Home Remedies* (listed in the reference section) are books which outline hydrotherapy treatments as well as other natural healing methods.

EXERCISE /3-C PRINCIPLE

There is no way around it: It would be very difficult to recover from Candida without following a proper exercise program. Because all components of the 3-C Program work together to facilitate recovery, it would be difficult to list them in order of importance. Exercise is just as vital as what one eats when trying to recover from Candida and other illnesses. Exercise provides many benefits, such as strengthening the heart and the other involuntary muscles (such as the stomach, uterus, and intestines) while reducing blood pressure and stress, slowing down the aging process (thus helping the body to look and feel younger), and reducing the risk of all degenerative diseases (such as arthritis, osteoporosis, and cancer). However, there are additional, less well-known benefits of exercise that are exceptionally significant in battling Candida, including:

—All illnesses have a more difficult time surviving in an oxygen base. Exercise promotes deep breathing, which brings more oxygen into the body, discouraging illness.

—Exercise helps the digestive system work more efficiently, resulting in fewer allergic reactions. Experience has shown that those who exercise properly will more quickly be able to tolerate foods and chemicals they have previously been allergic to.

—Exercise helps *immeasurably* to balance the low blood sugar symptoms that affect nearly all Candida patients. In particular, sustained exercise early in the day produces hormones that have multiple benefits. Combined with a consistent diet of whole foods (with no eating between meals), exercise regulates the blood sugar level throughout the entire day. This benefit alone can help eliminate many symptoms, including depression, fatigue, and confusion.

—Exercise curbs the appetite, which will help in the beginning of the 3-C Program, especially if a person is accustomed to several meals a day.

—Exercise facilitates the release of toxins, which is especially useful in the first few weeks of the 3-C Program. As a person begins taking *Kyolic* liquid garlic (See Chapter 5, 3-C Helpers) and following the 3-C Diet, the body will experience considerable cleansing, typically referred to as die-off. Processing and eliminating these additional toxins are burdensome to several organs of the body, since they are already processing normal body wastes. Exercise helps the body rid itself of these extra toxins through perspiration.

—Exercise helps to balance the thyroid and, therefore, metabolism. This, in turn, strengthens the immune system.

—Exercise is extremely beneficial in alleviating physical and mental stress.

What Type of Exercise Is Best?

When dealing with exercise, it is important to understand that maximum benefits can be realized only if exercise is used properly. Stressing the importance of exercise in the 3-C Program often elicits comments such as: "I'm active all day at my job," or, "I chase after a two-year-old. Why would I need more exercise?" Please realize that there is a difference between just being active and sustained exercise. "Being active" is usually a stop-and-go condition. For instance, mopping the floor can be a strenuous activity until it is interrupted by answering the phone or the door, which results in a drop in the heart rate. In order for an exercise program to be effective, it must consist of an aerobic exercise that will force the heart and lungs to work *long enough*, not just hard enough. Although endurance and muscular strength are healthy attributes, *sustained exercise produces additional vital benefits for candida patients that are not derived from any other component of the 3-C Program.*

Many fitness plans, as well as some experts, advise three, 30-minute sessions per week as a proper exercise program. That may be adequate for those who are simply interested in improving their cardiovascular health or body condition. However, for those who are trying to recover from a serious illness and desire more than these commonly-associated benefits, exercising *every single day* is absolutely necessary. After making measurable progress, some people have tried eliminating exercise only to find adverse symptoms (such as low blood sugar symptoms and/or allergies) returning. The importance of daily exercise, properly executed, cannot be over-emphasized.

Weight lifting, tennis, and calisthenics are fine to improve physical fitness; however, they are not considered sustained exercises. A sustained activity such as brisk walking, cycling, or low-impact aerobics is necessary in the 3-C Program. Walking is ideal since it offers the least amount of equipment investment, can be accomplished by anyone regardless of age, and has shown a low number of associated injuries. If walking is out of the question, because of unsafe neighborhoods, extremely cold weather, or poor walking surfaces, then an alternative exercise can be chosen.

It may be necessary to experiment with various types of exercise until one is found that is satisfactory. Regardless of what exercise is employed, a proper exercise program must include all three phases described below, and it should be enjoyable! Statistics show that choosing the right exercise is the key to perseverance. For example, some people may dislike aerobic dancing classes because they feel uncoordinated and self-conscious in front of others. They might feel more comfortable walking. Others would rather stay at home and follow various exercise programs on video or television. A little patience may be required until a preferred exercise is found. Also remember that most people do not immediately love exercise, especially when they don't feel well. However, be assured that the body will eventually respond with very positive mental, as well as physical, benefits.

Proper Exercise Cycles

Beginning any exercise regimen requires a healthy dose of common sense. It is always wise to check with a doctor or health professional before initiating an exercise plan. Although walking is used as an example below because it is an exercise that anyone can do, remember that any exercise can be utilized in this program as long as it is a three-phase, 60-minute, continuous program.

PHASE ONE – WARM UP - 20 Minutes

Start walking at a normal pace, increasing it gradually every few minutes. By the end of the first 20 minutes, a very brisk walking pace should be reached. Remember to swing arms at about the same pace.

PHASE TWO – PEAK PHASE - *20 Minutes*

Maintain this very brisk walking pace, which should be just short of jogging. Walk as fast as possible, swinging arms and pushing for perspiration during this entire phase.

PHASE THREE – COOL DOWN - *20 Minutes*

This phase should be the reverse of the first phase, every few minutes decreasing from a very brisk walking pace to a normal walking pace. It is especially important that the warm-up and cool-down phases be very gradual, so the heart is not overexerted.

If it is physically impossible to start with a full 60-minute workout, then one of shorter duration, based on capability, is advised. Add one or two more minutes each day, gradually building up to the full 60 minutes. Regardless of the length of the initial workout, always divide that time into the recommended three phases. For example, if the initial workout consists of 15 minutes, it should be divided into three five-minute phases. Keep in mind that exercise time should be uninterrupted. If unavoidably interrupted, at least keep moving the feet or arms at the appropriate rate.

It is possible to combine several different forms of exercise for variety. For example, an indoor program could begin the "warm-up phase" with stretching and jumping on a mini-trampoline. The "peak phase" could be a workout including a stationary bicycle or an aerobic video. (Some video exercise programs include warm-up and cool-down phases.) The "cool-down" phase could be the reverse of the warm-up phase, such as jumping on a mini-trampoline and, finally, stretching. Just remember not to stop between phases.

It is important to breathe deeply when exercising, in through the nose and out through the mouth. This is essential, whether exercising in or out-of-doors. Some people may experience pain in their side when exercising. This is most typically caused by taking in more oxygen than is expelled. A good way to avoid this is to breathe out for a longer count than you breathe in. For example, inhale for four counts and exhale for seven or eight counts.

WHEN TO EXERCISE

It is *strongly* recommended that exercise take place early in the morning! It may be difficult at first to get out of bed early if one is not normally an early riser. It may be necessary to summon forth multitudes of will power, especially for those who are chronically fatigued. However, exercising early in the morning is definitely superior to any other time of day for those recovering from Candida. According to several research studies, certain hormones in the blood are more abundant in the early morning hours. These "activity" hormones are responsible for: stabilizing blood sugar levels, strengthening the immune system, helping to digest food, alleviating allergies, and producing energy. In other words, these hormones are those that help one begin an active, productive day as well as function better throughout the rest of the day. At no other time during the day are they at such high levels. Exercising during this time further increases these levels so that Candida patients can take advantage of these excellent benefits.

If it is absolutely impossible to exercise early in the morning, then establish a regular exercise time either mid-morning, mid-afternoon, or early evening, keeping in mind that regularity is a crucial factor. Make sure to exercise at the same time every day, and make sure it is at least two hours after eating. It is also a good idea not to eat for at least 20 minutes after exercising. Heavy exercise either immediately before or after a meal will **delay** the digestion process. Mild exercise (such as gardening, shopping, and cleaning), however, promotes digestion.

Exercise Clothing And Shoes

Exercise clothing should be loose-fitting and comfortable. Cotton is ideal because it breathes. Clothing absorbs toxins from perspiration, so clothing should be removed promptly after exercising and laundered frequently. Clothing with tight waist, arm, or leg bands that may restrict movement and circulation should be avoided. To prevent the body from reabsorbing toxins, showers or baths immediately after exercising are recommended. Sufficient layers of clothing should be worn to prevent chilling. The entire body should be kept evenly covered so there are no differences in temperature, which affect circulation and the immune system. For this reason, it is important to keep the hands, head, and feet as warm as the rest of the body, not only during exercise, but at all times.

Investing in a pair of good quality exercise shoes will go a long way towards making an exercise program enjoyable. A reputable store with knowledgeable salespeople can provide the proper shoes for each person and her or his chosen exercise. Especially in walking, jogging, or aerobics, this is very important. Shoes should be fitted allowing enough room to accommodate cotton sports socks, which will absorb moisture during exercise. Shoes should be thoroughly aired out before the next use.

Statistics show that half of those starting an exercise program will not continue for more than a few months. It may be that those who feel more in control of their lives and have a higher self-esteem tend to have a better attitude regarding exercise. Rather than viewing exercise as something they have to do, they see it as another avenue to improve who they are, much like an education or a promotion. Unfortunately, many Candida patients cringe at the very thought of exercise. For them, viewing exercise as one of the tools necessary for recovery may be more difficult. The bottom line is that it may take some time to reach the point when exercise becomes enjoyable, but the vital benefits to Candida patients are well worth it.

AIR/3-C PRINCIPLE

Being outside in the fresh air every day is a healthy habit that most people neglect, yet is a valuable asset in the 3-C Program. Air is made up of both positive and negative ions; negative ions are the most beneficial. They are nourishing to the respiratory and immune systems. Although negative ions can be in all homes in small quantities, they are found in abundance in nature, especially near water, trees, and sunlight. It is ideal to allow as much natural air into the home as possible every day, especially into the bedrooms. If possible, bedroom windows should be kept open just a crack, even in cool weather, but direct drafts should be avoided. Morning is a good time to throw back the covers on the bed and let the fresh air and sunlight absorb toxins from the bedclothes.

One factor that contributes to many of today's degenerative diseases is a lack of fresh air. People working in "airtight" buildings would benefit from stepping outside during breaks and breathing fresh air deeply for five to ten minutes. It may be surprising how refreshing these short breaks can be.

SUNLIGHT/*3-C PRINCIPLE*

For the most part, modern Americans have neglected to take advantage of one of the best natural healers in the environment — the sun! However, Europeans have traditionally recognized the health benefits of sunshine. One of their long-standing habits is to place items such as mattresses and bed-clothing in the sun. They also realize the sun can keep people healthy, and that is why spending time outside is more a part of their routine.

When exposed to the ultraviolet light in natural sunshine, the body produces more white blood cells, particularly lymphocytes, necessary to fight infection and protect against disease. In fact, in 1903, a Nobel prize was awarded for successful treatment of tuberculosis through the use of ultraviolet light. The nerve endings under the skin actually trap energy from the sun and transmit it down into the cells and organs of the body. Dr. Zane Kime, in his book *Sunlight*, says ultraviolet light from the sun can benefit the entire body. Below are some of these benefits:

ULTRAVIOLET LIGHT CAN:

Raise
Body's resistance to
  infections
Oxygen-carrying capacity
  of blood
Adrenalin in tissues
Tolerance to stress
Sex hormone levels
Resistance to skin infections
Energy, endurance, and
  muscular strength

Lower
Blood pressure
Resting heart rate
Blood cholesterol
Glycogen stores in liver
Blood sugar

Just as regular exercise can boost the immune system, so can regular, limited exposure to the sun. Also, the sun promotes the production of Vitamin D. Because the Vitamin D requirements of humans cannot be met through food alone (both the animal and plant kingdom are deficient), perhaps nature intended for us to obtain Vitamin D from the sun all along.

The sun converts components in the skin into pre-Vitamin D, which is then converted to Vitamin D via body heat. This conversion process is also thought to encourage the formation of healthy hormones, much like exercise does. Especially important for Candida patients is the fact that even a few minutes of sunlight can help move sugar from the blood to the liver, helping to stabilize blood sugar. The sun also encourages the thyroid to increase hormones, which in turn increases metabolism, burning more calories. The sun helps to provide not only essential Vitamin D, but also the extra calming effect produced by the calcium absorption that Vitamin D triggers. In today's world, who doesn't need a good dose of that?

Of course, everyone is concerned about the connection between sunlight and skin cancer. While it is possible to expose the body to too much sunlight, Dr. Kime feels that skin cancer is more likely connected to other factors:

—The typical American diet as explained in Chapter 3, fats and a general lack of nutrients in today's diet pose problems for many reasons, but these are multiplied when combined with sunlight. Ultraviolet light from the sun, acting on the high polyunsaturated triglycerides in the blood from a high-fat diet, increases the chance of skin cancer. Burning of the skin plus the use of polyunsaturated fat accelerates this process and weakens the immune system. In fact, polyunsaturated fat so greatly inhibits the immune system that its use is specifically included in the diet of kidney transplant patients so their bodies will be less likely to reject foreign tissue. Therefore, while constant exposure to or repeated burning from the sun may contribute to skin cancer, sunlight in itself does not cause cancer. Diet is actually more of a contributing factor to skin cancer than sunlight.

—The use of oils and creams on the skin. The dangers of fat are not restricted to food. Externally applied compounds are also very likely to be rancid, causing free radical formation that can contribute to cancer (see Chapter 3, Limit Refined Or Concentrated Foods). For example, sunscreens that contain para-aminobenzoic acid (PABA) are supposed to protect from the sun. However, Dr. Kime points out that research now shows that PABA can cause genetic damage when exposed to sunlight. Think of the repercussions of this! PABA is contained in hundreds of cosmetics, lotions, and sunscreens. How ironic that sunscreens are used to prevent burning and cancer when actually they are contributing to the problem! In addition, Dr. Kime says suntan lotions will not promote tanning or prevent wrinkling of the skin.

—Serious over-exposure. Too much of even a good thing can be bad, and the same is true of the sun. While only a few minutes a day are necessary to benefit the immune system, spending a little more time in the sun is not dangerous if caution is used. Burning should never be allowed because it encourages free radical formation. It is interesting to note that studies show those consuming and using less fats in the diet do not burn nearly as easily. Once again, the diet makes the difference.

So, what can be done to lower skin-cancer risk? First of all, fat in the diet must be reduced. Second, showers should be taken before going out into the sun to remove soaps, lotions, powders, perfume, and powder residue which can cause skin to be more sensitive and burn more easily. Third, those with skin types that burn easily should simply take it slower and not stay in the sun as long. An added benefit of tanning slowly is it will give the skin a nice, soft appearance instead of the dried-out look that over-exposure produces.

Especially in the beginning of the 3-C Program, it is very healthful to actually sunbathe for a few minutes every day, if possible. Depending on skin type, it is wise to begin with only a few minutes and build up to at least 15 to 20 minutes every day. (Don't forget to turn over!) If actually "lying" in the sun is not possible, try to at least spend as much time as possible in the sun. Tanning beds are not recommended since they do not provide the full spectrum of natural light. Too much ultraviolet light alone may actually break the chromosomes in the cells of the body.

Research shows that as little as 15 minutes per day of sunlight through the eyes or on the face can supply one with adequate amounts of Vitamin D. Caution: Do not go outside and look directly at the sun. Simply go outside without glasses or contact lenses and sit or work in the sunshine.

Those who work inside all day should make it a practice to go out into the natural light several times a day. Eating lunch outdoors or taking a walk is ideal. Benefits can be derived from changing indoor lighting from fluorescent and/or incandescent, which are damaging to the immune system, to a type of lighting called full spectrum. This lighting more closely resembles natural light and has been credited with improving problems ranging from headaches to hyperactivity. Full spectrum lighting used to be rather expensive, but there are now more suppliers offering these lights at a reasonable cost.

With a little common sense, the natural healing benefits of the sun can be taken advantage of. Dr. Kime's book is an excellent source of information regarding the true causes of skin cancer. (See Reference section.) Unfortunately, modern theory is discouraging the use of one of the immune system's best friends by claiming its link to cancer. Is the sun really an enemy? Obviously, previous generations did not think so, since they spent a good deal of their life working outside and were not plagued with skin cancer. Has the sun changed since then? No, but diets have! Skin cancer, as well as other illness, is a disease brought on by modern man, not the sun.

REST /3-C PRINCIPLE

Many people are aware of the importance of a good night's rest, but the benefits of a proper sleep schedule are not widely known. Not only does sleep replenish the supply of energy, it actually encourages rebuilding of the entire body! Because many of the body systems slow down during periods of rest (the central nervous system is almost entirely suspended), the body has time to repair and reproduce vital cells while shedding toxins. There is just no substitute for this rebuilding process, which occurs more effectively because of certain hormones that can only be produced before midnight. *Therefore, the most beneficial sleep occurs in the hours before midnight.* In fact, many proponents of early sleep claim that the hours of sleep before midnight are twice as profitable to the body as those after midnight. Another important factor is that the body does not complete its healing cycle if sleep is constantly interrupted or if sleeping times are not long enough to include all stages of sleep. Therefore, a *continuous* sleep of seven to eight hours is best.

In order to obtain all the benefits of sleep, one must go without interruption through all five stages. These five stages are divided into two main categories called REM (Rapid Eye Movement) and NREM (Non Rapid Eye Movement). People sleep in cycles, going back and forth, in and out of these categories at least four or five times in an eight-hour night. During certain cycles, growth hormones are produced by the pituitary gland, which are important in the metabolic restorative process after a day's exertions.

REM sleep is so vital to human functioning that the body will make up for its loss during subsequent sleeping sessions. A person will normally have three to four sessions per night at 80 to 120-minute intervals, with each REM episode lasting from 5-60 minutes. In one experiment in a sleep lab, a subject was awakened each time he entered REM sleep. The first night he was awakened five times and on subsequent nights he was awakened more and more, until one night he had to be awakened 200 times. Finally the subject, upon going to sleep, went immediately into REM sleep and could not be awakened. Anything that overcomes REM sleep, like alcohol, drugs, and most sleeping medications, will create REM debt and make one pay interest until paid in full. Without REM sleep a person wakes up irritable, tired, depressed, angry, restless, and/or apathetic.

Contrary to what most people think, mornings are the most productive time for creative work, physical tasks, and eye/hand coordination. That's because hormones levels that promote these functions actually peak early in the morning, shortly before sunrise. These "activity" hormones are evidenced by measuring blood levels at various times during the day. Both the male and female hormone levels, which encourage active mind and body functions, are at their highest early in the day. These hormones help muscles to move and brains to think. They literally help the body to advance from a complete sedentary state to a functional "wide-awake" state. These same hormones assist the body in other functions as well, such as stabilizing blood sugar and producing enzymes that help digest food.

Conversely, evenings are a time to "wind down." Blood tests also reveal that shortly before sunset the body begins to increase the production of a hormone called melatonin. This hormone is responsible for producing a sleepy feeling. Sleep then encourages the production of a second hormone that is vital for repairing the body and promoting growth. The deeper the sleep, the more abundant this hormone. Therefore, it is not surprising that early bedtimes, as well as regular exercise, can stimulate the growth hormone, so important for a child's development.

Naturally, the body is better able to release enzymes and hormones when people cooperate with their natural biological time clock. Habits such as staying up very late and sleeping late the next morning interfere with this natural process, resulting in a person feeling groggy and hard-to-wake-up in the morning.

Many people insist they cannot possibly go to bed early because they either have too much to do in the evenings or they simply cannot fall asleep. These people have been functioning as "night owls" for so long that they have actually fooled their bodies into thinking this is a normal procedure. However, research studies have proven that once a schedule of "early to bed, early to rise" is established, productivity is actually higher in the morning hours!

Many people are overwhelmed by the demands of both working and taking care of a family. They usually rush home from work to fix dinner and spend the rest of the evening trying to "catch up" on housework or other tasks. Since the hormones responsible for physical energy and mental acuity are more abundant in the early morning hours, it is not surprising that studies show that a person can be nearly twice as productive early in the day as opposed to late in the day when "activity" hormones are decreasing and those that induce sleep are starting to rise. Many people have reported that they can accomplish more in two morning hours than in four evening hours. They also find that getting up ahead of everyone else allows them to organize their day and get off to a good start.

Although it may take up to 30 days to become accustomed to a new sleeping pattern, this can be initiated by simply forcing the body to get up at an earlier time. Avoid napping and use all of the 3-C principles to make going to bed early a welcomed experience. Remember that daily physical activity should be equal to or preferably greater than mental activity. Toxins in the body, especially during die-off, can irritate the nerves and cause insomnia. Exercise, as well as fresh air, help to reduce toxins and increase oxygen intake.

Other factors that can affect sleeping patterns are snacking or eating a large meal in the evening. If following the three-meal plan of the 3-C Program, make sure the third meal is eaten no later than 6 PM and equals no more than 10 to 20 percent of total intake for the day. The two-meal plan is preferable, because it allows ample time for the early stage of digestion to take place before going to bed. In this way, **delay** in the digestive system is avoided.

Napping

Many Candida patients are chronically tired and nap quite often. But napping will become a thing of the past shortly after implementing the 3-C Program. Keep in mind that the fatigue factor may not be reduced until after a good deal of die-off has transpired, then most people report abundant energy. Resisting the urge to nap is important for two reasons. First of all, lying down within two to three hours after a meal will **delay** the digestion process. Second, napping can interfere with healthy patterns of sleep, producing poor-quality sleep at night, resulting in tiredness the next day, leading to taking a nap, and so on. In other words, napping creates a vicious cycle that never seems to produce truly restful sleep.

The best way to energize oneself, if faced with the urge to nap, is to take a brisk walk outside in the fresh air. People are amazed how good they feel when only a few minutes earlier they were ready to fall asleep. Walking is certainly not the only "energizer." One 3-C Program participant related how she would put on her favorite record and dance all around the house. Another woman said that whenever she felt exhausted and tempted to go to bed, she would drop her work and do something that was fun or interesting to her, such as shopping, gardening, or visiting friends. Within a few minutes, she had forgotten how tired she was.

If it is not possible to go outside for a few minutes, resting upright in a comfortable chair for 10 to 15 minutes can be refreshing. Setting a kitchen timer or alarm will allow complete relaxation without worry about falling asleep. Even if it is necessary to force oneself to get moving when the alarm goes off, after rising most people feel energized enough to remain active until bedtime.

Bedtimes

When following the 3-C Program, the ideal schedule requires going to bed at 9:00 PM and rising at 5:00 AM. (See 3-C Schedule in Chapter 5.) This is especially important when trying to recover from an illness. If at all possible, do not deviate from this schedule, even if it becomes necessary to change work schedules or other routines. Participants in this program consistently find the sooner they adjust their regular bedtimes, the faster they recover. Remember, there is healing to be accomplished before midnight, and it is necessary to get as much sleep before then as possible. The "9 to 5" sleep schedule allows one hour in the morning to get things done before starting exercise. Most Candida patients find that this works out to be the ideal rising and retiring time.

If it is absolutely impossible to follow the 9 to 5 schedule, small deviations can be allowed. Going to bed at 9:30 PM and getting up at 5:30 AM may work just fine. However, going to bed later than 10:00 PM and getting up at 6:00 AM would leave very little time for exercise and a shower before eating breakfast at 7:00 AM. It is important not to postpone breakfast much past 7:00 AM because that will delay the entire day's schedule. As a result, those following the three-meal plan would be eating too late in the evening, possibly causing **delay** in the digestive process. Remember that five hours must be left between the end of one meal and the beginning of the next. On the two-meal plan, breakfast should be eaten no later than 7:30 AM. Chapter 5 contains an ideal schedule to follow for either of these plans.

REGULARITY/*3-C PRINCIPLE*

Even though regularity appears last on the 3-C Sign, its importance should not be underestimated. Especially during recovery, it is not only crucial to implement every component of the 3-C Program but to do so *regularly*. Most people do not realize that the body functions more efficiently on a regular basis. Research studies have proven there are observable, measurable rhythms of the mind and body known as biorhythms (not to be confused with the non-scientific fad that was popular several years ago).

Scientific biorhythm study is based on multitudes of observable periodic phenomena. It is the science of Chronobiology, which allows the measuring and documentation of actual biorhythms. True biorhythms exist on a daily, weekly, monthly, yearly, and seasonal basis. Circadian rhythms, which occur in 24-hour cycles, probably impact people the most. These are the rhythms which seem to correlate with the hormone production of the body, which reveals at what times during the day the body is more capable of performing certain tasks. A professor from the University of Massachusetts, Dr. John Palmer, says, "Because of the living clock's relentless activity, we are not the same person from one hour to the next; but at the *same time each day, we are much like we were the day before and much like we will be tomorrow.*" Obviously, people more proficiently perform functions such as eating, sleeping, supplying energy, and digesting food on a regular, rhythmical basis. The following is an example of the impact of biorhythms, demonstrated by studying their correlation with eating:

—Shortly before waking, the digestive juices are stirring, due to an increase of chloride in the blood. Chloride helps to produce stomach acids and the enzyme amylase, which is very necessary in the digestive process. Chloride is at its highest level very early in the day.

—The body also provides an abundance of enzymes and amino acids that help break down protein early in the day. For example, protein eaten by 4:00 PM is better utilized than protein eaten later in the day. Likewise, meals eaten later in the evening can cause a **delay** in the digestion process of up to 12 hours because protein is especially difficult to digest while sleeping. Eating the majority of protein earlier in the day supplies energy. On the other hand, eating protein late in the day results in fat production for two reasons. First, levels of insulin and glucose are highest in the late afternoon, which encourages fat formation; and second very little energy is used after eating an evening meal before one goes to bed. No wonder many people who are dieting are frustrated after reducing their overall daily caloric intake and they are still not losing weight. They are probably eating the largest percentage of their daily food supply in the late afternoon and evening.

—Iron production, which provides energy, is also affected by eating habits. When eating earlier meals, iron levels will peak at approximately 7:00 AM and remain at a more constant supply throughout the late afternoon, when people need energy the most. Eating later, such as skipping breakfast or lunch, will stall iron production until late afternoon or early evening. Once again, a short-change of energy occurs during the day when it is really needed.

—Since hypoglycemia symptoms are so prevalent in Candida patients, it is important to understand that eating early in the morning is essential. Blood sugar levels are typically low for everyone in the mornings, regardless of how much was eaten, or how late, the previous evening. Therefore, eating in the evenings does not stabilize low blood sugar. Instead, eating early in the day provides the body with the substance it needs to stabilize the blood sugar. Regular exercise, regular eating times, and a proper diet will adequately stabilize blood sugar and energy levels. Conversely, a lack of exercise, irregular eating schedules, and a poor diet encourage low blood sugar. (See Chapter 8, Hypoglycemia.)

It should now be apparent that the proper timing of meals is just as important as what is eaten. This is true not only in eating but in every component of the 3-C Program, including sleeping, exercising, and drinking water. Unfortunately, today's lifestyles frequently are in opposition to the natural biological time clock. Eating patterns, sleeping patterns, the state of the environment, diet, and travel are just a few elements that can throw natural rhythms out of sync. For this reason, a regular schedule is crucial when initiating the 3-C Program. It will actually assist in rebalancing the body's natural biorhythms and promote recovery.

Stress

Even though stress is not a main component of the 3-C Program, it has a definite effect on overall health, specifically the immune system. In today's world, too much stress can be a result of juggling multiple roles/functions and coping with the daily changes and dilemmas that occur within these roles/functions. Unfortunately, it is even becoming popular to be "stressed out." A common misconception is that unless one is stressed out, she or he is not working hard enough.

Stress is one of the many factors that contribute to the breakdown of an immune system, and it must be dealt with. Stress can adversely affect the recovery of a Candida patient. In a few isolated cases, positive results from the 3-C Program were limited until the subject of stress was addressed. For example, if a Candida patient has been faithfully following the program and there is no apparent physical reason for a lack of progress or a sudden setback, stress can often be blamed. Many times people are not even aware of a source of stress in their lives until a thorough investigation is made. Once the source of stress is identified and dealt with, Candida patients can continue their progress.

Physical Reactions To Stress

Physical reactions to stress are either short-term or long-term. Short-term stress is characterized by a series of rapid physical reactions to alleviate the stressful situation. The heart races, blood pressure builds, and blood surges to the muscles. Oxygen and extra nutrients are sent to the brain to increase alertness. The secretion of adrenaline is also increased. These physical responses play a part in **delaying** the digestion process. Trying to cope with the effects of stress on other parts of the body takes energy away from the digestive process. For this reason one should strive to make mealtimes as pleasant as possible.

When stress is long-term (marriage, job, family problem), a series of hormonal reactions take place, culminating in the release of a hormone called cortisol from the adrenal glands. While cortisol increases blood sugar and speeds up metabolism, it also suppresses the immune system. These changes, while beneficial for a short-term emergency such as providing super-strength in a crisis situation, are actually harmful when produced on a continual basis.

Stress is said to be one of the most powerful factors affecting the immune system. Extensive research over the last ten years has shown that the mind can and does exert a real, biochemical influence on the body. For example, the trauma of losing a spouse is rated as one of the most stressful situations in life. Surviving spouses consistently show suppressed immune-system response. In fact, the mortality rate among surviving spouses during the first year after their mate's death is two to six times higher than the average.

Coping With Stress Mentally And Physically

Coping with stress takes time, patience, and honesty. First, it is necessary to identify the stressful situations (stressors) in one's life. Make a list of all the stressful situations or persons who are a source of stress, no matter how insignificant. Put an "A" next to those stressors that, with a little thought and effort, could be resolved. Even though these small stressors are more easily managed, they often go unrecognized. Combined, they can cause more stress than realized. Situations such as having to rush to daycare in order to pick up children on time every day creates a stressful situation for all. Or perhaps one has a dog but has no time to spend with it, complaining about having to feed it and let it out, yet doing nothing to remedy the situation. Since dealing with the sum total of all of these little stressors in a person's life can be exhausting physically and mentally, it is important to make changes. For example, arrange for someone else to pick up the children from daycare. Find someone who would give the dog the attention it deserves.

The remaining stressors should be marked "B," and consist of conditions or people who create situations over which one has less control. Any ideas that will aid in coping with stressors on list "B" should be written next to them. Although many times there is little one can do to correct a situation, changing one's attitude regarding it can, in itself, relieve some stress. In these instances, focusing on acceptance and coping techniques may be the only option. For example, if a person has a friend or relative who is a constant source of conflict, and all attempts to reason with him or her provide no results, it will do no good to continue arguing. Instead, avoiding arguements, compromising more often, or simply avoiding this person would be less stressful for all. Constantly agonizing over a situation creates the long-term type of stress that can weaken the immune system. Coping and acceptance techniques can be facilitated by other resources, such as friends, professionals, clergy, or literature. Also, remember that one of the best stress-relievers is exercise, which strengthens the body mentally, as well as physically.

This chapter has focused on the importance of making proper lifestyle choices based on a regular schedule, which brings to mind the lifestyles of previous generations. They were part of a more orderly, rural, agrarian society (rather than a stressful, driven, global society) that dictated healthy lifestyle habits such as eating a good diet, performing most physical labor in the sun and fresh air, and drinking better quality water. In addition, they performed all of these healthy lifestyles on a regular schedule. Even though it may not be possible to revert to lifestyles that were common 50 years ago, it is possible to make lifestyle choices that work with, rather than against, the natural biological time clock. These practices strengthen the immune system, helping to prevent degenerative diseases.

PRINCIPLES THAT REGULATE THE DIGESTIVE SYSTEM

Chew Food Well
Eat Two Or Three Meals A Day With Nothing Between
Liquids Should Not Be Consumed With Meals
Eliminate Eating In The Evenings
Reduce Number Of Foods At Each Meal
Practice Simple Food Combining
Limit Refined And Concentrated Foods
Utilize Proper Exercise At Proper Times
Control Stress

CHAPTER 5

GETTING WELL

The 3-C Program is divided into two segments, "Getting Well" and "Staying Well." This book focuses mainly on Getting Well since the first priority is to recover from poor health. Once Candida or other negative symptoms have subsided, there are certain flexibilities allowed, such as additions to diet and variations in exercise times, that will be discussed in Chapter 7, Staying Well. Naturally, many people are curious as to how long the Getting Well segment of this program will take. Since varying, multiple factors contribute to a person's state of illness, it would be very difficult to predict the time it takes to recover. Naturally, the more extensive the damage to the immune system, the longer it will take to repair that damage.

Implementing the 3-C Program properly usually brings relief from symptoms in approximately 30 to 60 days. In other words, most recovering Candida patients find relief from symptoms such as allergic reactions, low blood sugar, and chronic fatigue within the first few weeks; however, more stubborn conditions may take a few months longer. Even though Candida patients are eager to recover, it is crucial to allow the immune system the time it needs to totally complete the healing process, however long that may be. The important point is that when Candida patients implement the 3-C Program, they begin to feel better in a matter of weeks and months, compared to possibly years of illness.

The Body Responds To Lifestyle Changes

After practicing poor lifestyle choices for years without apparent ill effects, Candida patients may be a little confused to find their immune system suddenly crumbling. They may not be aware that the immune system is truly a wonder of nature that has the ability to tolerate multiple poor-lifestyle habits — up to a point. Eventually, the immune system encounters that one factor, or group of factors, that constitutes the "straw that broke the camel's back." Fortunately, the immune system has the ability to recover when proper lifestyle choices are made.

Withdrawal, Detoxification, and Die-Off

Withdrawal, detoxification, and die-off are processes that take place, to some degree, for nearly every Candida patient. Some people may be aware of it and some may not. As favorable lifestyle choices replace poor ones, the body naturally eliminates toxins that may have been accumulating for years. Even though the term "withdrawal" is commonly associated with the abrupt discontinuation of vices such as drugs, alcohol, or cigarettes, withdrawal can also occur due to the discontinuation of harmful substances from other everyday sources. Chemicals used to enhance, preserve, and flavor food and water; hormones and antibiotics used in animal products; drug medications, and many other foreign substances can accumulate in the body. No wonder withdrawal is experienced when instituting a new diet, beginning regular exercise, and incorporating other positive lifestyle changes!

As a reaction to the withdrawal of undesirable substances, the immune system, accustomed to defending the body against harmful substances, begins to eliminate these accumulated toxins. This "detoxification" is the immune system's way of cleaning house. Just as bothersome dust is sometimes raised when cleaning house, some unpleasant experiences may occur in the body when the 3-C Program is begun. One or more symptoms of detoxification, such as irritability, sleeplessness, joint and muscle pains, lethargy, headaches, or skin problems may appear.

Kyolic liquid garlic is employed in the 3-C Program to rebuild the immune system, and it may also produce detoxification. This garlic has the ability to stimulate and strengthen the immune system so it can combat and reduce yeast overgrowth on its own. As the yeast in the body is reduced (or "dies" as is typically said), the residue is thrown into the bloodstream for elimination, causing more detoxification. One or more symptoms may occur as a result of this "die-off" reaction. These can be similar to the detoxification symptoms previously described, or may actually appear as a worsening of a Candida patient's original symptoms.

Between detoxification and die-off symptoms, it can be common for a person to feel as though she (or he) is actually regressing instead of progressing. *Do not be discouraged.* Healing the body is like the peeling of an onion, layer by layer. Accumulated toxins or residues of previous illnesses may temporarily resurface, once again producing familiar symptoms. For example, one man who had rheumatic fever as a child experienced a one-day recurrence of symptoms similar to those of the original illness. Although this does not always occur, it is possible to experience a "mini-version" of previous illnesses during detoxification. Sometimes referred to as a "healing crisis," this is usually nothing to be alarmed about. It is a normal, eliminative function of the immune system. Just as a physician cannot set a broken bone without some pain, attaining good health is usually not possible without the discomfort of accumulated toxins being cleansed from the body.

Keep in mind that many Candida patients report increased energy and improvement from the very beginning of the program. Others may experience some degree of detoxification or die-off, the duration of which will be dependent on prior states of health, the amount of Candida in the body, and how much *Kyolic* liquid garlic is taken. It is wise to start slowly when taking *Kyolic* liquid garlic and build up as tolerance allows. If larger doses of *Kyolic* liquid garlic are used initially, detoxification may be so severe it would be difficult to adhere to the recommended daily schedule. For instance, if a person feels too "wiped out" to exercise, detoxing is happening too quickly. Guidelines are given for *Kyolic* liquid garlic doses later in this chapter under "3-C Helpers."

Most people move through the majority of detoxification or die-off in a few weeks. Experience has shown that if a person exercises properly, keeps active throughout the day, and drinks plenty of water, die-off symptoms are much more tolerable. Whether or not a person experiences detoxification or die-off symptoms is not important. Either way, recovery will occur with patience and perseverance.

One of the keys to recovery from illness is attitude. For instance, if a person has been on a typical American diet, the 3-C Diet will be a challenge. It involves cooking with different foods using different methods. Patience and perseverance, coupled with a good attitude, will help a person view these changes as *choices* toward recovery. If people should ever feel the effort is not worth it, they need only to ask themselves how much they want to overcome their health problems. If they are tired of their state of health and the restrictions it has placed on their life, they need to make a decision. Do they want disease to continue to control their life or not? *Choice* is the key word. With many illnesses, people can choose health or "unhealth." If they choose to get well, then it should be reflected in their attitude as well as their actions. Instead of sitting back begrudgingly and waiting for this program to work, they should anticipate positive results. Instead of looking for others to support them, they should be their own biggest supporter. They should be thankful that God, with His bountiful nature, has provided the knowledge and necessary foods to rebuild the body naturally.

THE 3-C SCHEDULE

Through the media, doctors, health professionals, and groups such as the American Heart Association and the American Cancer Society, Americans have come to grips with the fact that diet and other lifestyle factors can definitely make a difference in one's state of health. However, there are other lifestyle changes not recognized by most health authorities that can promote recovery from Candida and other illness.

As discussed previously, the human body functions better if it knows *what to expect* and *when to expect it*. This is especially true during recovery! Many people either interrupt their recovery or never really make progress because they do not recognize the importance of regularity in their lifestyle. To avoid this interruption or lack of progress, it is necessary not only to implement all of the lifestyle principles of the

3-C Program but to do so on a regular basis. Otherwise, experience has shown that recovery may not be complete. *In other words, the degree of recovery is often in direct correlation to the degree to which the program is followed.*

In order to ensure that one includes all lifestyle principles in his or her daily schedule, it is imperative that one of the meal plan schedules be strictly followed. Even though a schedule may seem restricting at first, it assists one in setting aside a time for all components of the program, such as leaving enough time between meals, drinking adequate water, and so forth. If it is *absolutely impossible* to follow one of these schedules exactly, one should make as few variations as possible. Making these variations will be discussed later.

Because a major goal of the 3-C Program is to restore the immune system through the regulation of the digestive system, it only makes sense to base lifestyle principles around the digestive system and process. It is imperative for Candida patients to realize that every time a person eats, the digestion process is initiated. Merely emptying food from the stomach into the intestines is a taxing process that requires most often four to five hours. If this stage of digestion is interrupted, this process can be **delayed** for hours longer. (See Chapter 3.) Since digestion depletes the energy reserves of the body, eating only two meals per day, instead of three, will allow the digestive system additional time to rest and heal. The result is more overall energy and a more rapid recovery. Therefore, the two-meal plan is highly recommended.

There are some instances which would permit three meals per day. These include serious cravings, the need to eat often due to hypoglycemia, or being underweight. (Other suggestions for these conditions appear in Chapter 8.) Under these circumstances, it may be necessary to start with the three-meal plan. Keep in mind that following the 3-C Diet and simply giving the body time to benefit from this new schedule will help to curb cravings and balance energy. Whichever plan is chosen, the important thing to remember is to *be consistent.* Eating two meals one day and three the next will not provide the digestive system with the regularity it needs to recover. Once one has chosen a plan, stick with it for some time. Then, if for some reason, such as employment demands, one has to switch to a different meal plan, again, stick with it and do not flip back and forth from two to three meals.

TWO MEAL SCHEDULE

5:00 AM - Wake up and dress in exercise clothes. Drink at least two 8-oz. glasses of water. (See Chapter 4, Water Requirements.) May add the juice of one-half lemon to the morning water *only*. Assemble all items for the first meal.

5:30 AM - Begin exercise program as described in Chapter 4, Exercise. Exercise for a full, continuous 60 minutes.

6:30 AM - Return from exercise, take a quick shower, and prepare first meal.

7:00 AM - Prepare and drink digestive drink, carefully following instructions in the recipe section. (Add 3-C Helpers, such as *Kyolic* liquid garlic, *Kyo-Green* or psyllium seed, to the digestive drink.) Immediately eat first meal, taking acidophilus at end of meal with a few bites of food.

7:40 AM - Finish first meal. In order to aid digestion, keep lightly active after meals.

8:40 AM - May begin drinking water again. Most of daily water requirement should be consumed by late afternoon or early evening so that a good night's sleep is not interrupted by frequent trips to the bathroom. (See Chapter 4, Water Requirements.)

Journal Entry - Sometime during late morning, record physical state upon rising this morning, what was eaten at the first meal, amounts of 3-C Helpers taken, and physical state since eating the first meal. Note any reactions, fatigue, etc.

Sometime this morning, take a "sunshine and fresh air" break for 10-15 minutes, breathing deeply.

1:30 PM - Discontinue drinking water. Start to prepare second meal.

2:00 PM - Prepare and drink digestive drink, carefully following instructions in the recipe section. (Add *Kyolic* liquid garlic only to the digestive drink. *Kyo-Green* and psyllium seed need only be taken once a day.) Immediately eat second meal, taking acidophilus at end of meal with a few bites of food.

2:40 PM - Finish second meal. In order to aid digestion, keep lightly active after meals.

3:40 PM - May now begin drinking water again. Make sure to drink all water left in jug prior to 7:00 PM.

Sometime this afternoon, take a "sunshine and fresh air" break for 10-15 minutes, breathing deeply.

Journal Entry - Sometime during early evening, record what was eaten for the second meal, amounts of 3-C Helpers taken, and physical state. Note any reactions, fatigue, etc.

Check menu planner for the next day's meals.

9:00 PM - Bedtime

THREE MEAL SCHEDULE

5:00 AM - Wake up and dress in exercise clothes. Drink at least two 8-oz. glasses of water. (See Chapter 4, Water Requirements.) May add the juice of one-half lemon to the morning water *only*. Assemble all items for first meal.

5:15 AM - Begin exercise program as described in Chapter 4, Exercise. Exercise for a full, continuous 60 minutes.

6:15 AM - Return from exercise, take a quick shower and prepare first meal.

6:45 AM - Prepare and drink digestive drink, carefully following instructions in the recipe section. (Add 3-C Helpers, such as *Kyolic* liquid garlic, *Kyo-Green* or psyllium seed, to the digestive drink. Immediately eat first meal, taking acidophilus at the end of the meal with a few bites of food.

7:30 AM - Finish first meal. In order to aid digestion, keep lightly active after meals.

8:30 AM - May now begin drinking water again. Most of the daily water requirement should be consumed by 5:30 PM. By not drinking too much water later in the evening, a good night's sleep is not interrupted by frequent trips to the bathroom.

Journal Entry - Sometime during late morning, record physical state upon rising this morning, what was eaten at the first meal, amounts of 3-C Helpers taken, and physical state since eating the first meal. Note any reactions, fatigue, etc.

Sometime this morning, take a "sunshine and fresh air" break for 10-15 minutes, breathing deeply.

12:00 NOON - Discontinue drinking water. Start to prepare second meal.

12:30 PM - Prepare and drink digestive drink, carefully following instructions in the recipe section. (Add *Kyolic* liquid garlic only to the digestive drink. *Kyo Green* and psyllium seed need only be taken once a day.) Immediately eat second meal, taking acidophilus at end of meal with a few bites of food.

1:10 PM - Finish second meal. In order to aid digestion, keep lightly active after meals.

2:10 PM - May now begin drinking water again. Remember to drink all or nearly all water in the jug by 5:30 PM.

Sometime this afternoon, take a "sunshine and fresh air" break for 10 to 15 minutes, breathing deeply.

5:30 PM - Discontinue drinking water. Start to prepare third meal.

6:00 PM - Eat a light, third meal of only whole grains and/or one of the Exception Foods listed in Chapter 5. *It is not necessary to drink cabbage juice or take 3-C Helpers with the third meal.*

6:20 PM - Finish third meal. In order to aid digestion, keep lightly active after meals. Wait at least one hour to drink any water left in the jug. (There should be only a very small amount of water, if any, left.)

Journal Entry - During the evening, record what was eaten at the second and third meals, 3-C Helpers taken with second meal, and physical state since the last journal entry. Note any reactions, fatigue, etc.

Check menu planner for next day's meals.

9:00 PM - Bedtime

More About Schedules

Since initiating the 3-C Schedule and diet at the same time may seem a little overwhelming, it is often easier to start the Getting Well segment of this program in two phases. The first week, follow the 3-C Schedule only excluding the diet. Even though the 3-C Diet will not be put into action at this point, this period will help in adjusting to regular times of exercising, eating, drinking water, rising, and retiring. Use this week also to try new recipes and cooking methods, stocking the freezer with beans, whole grains, and grain items.

This is an ideal time to check with local suppliers for unfamiliar foods, purchase groceries, gather cooking utensils, and compose menus for the next few weeks. (Guidelines on these suggestions are given in Chapter 6.) The second phase of Getting Well is simply to incorporate the recommended 3-C Diet and to keep a journal, which are both discussed later in this chapter.

Keep in mind that making multiple changes in habits, schedules, and diet does not go unnoticed by the body. Below are some situations that may be encountered and tips on dealing with them:

Cravings- Since many Candida patients have been accustomed to eating quite often during the day, eating only two or three meals may cause them to experience cravings, hunger, or hypoglycemia-like symptoms in the beginning of the program. If these symptoms are severe during the first week of the program while not implementing the 3-C Diet, it may be necessary to go ahead and include at least beans in the diet to help stabilize blood sugar levels.

When following the two-meal plan in the beginning of the program, some Candida patients feel they cannot wait until 2:00 PM for their second meal. Although it is possible to eat earlier (five hours after finishing the first meal would be 12:40 PM), it will then be necessary to wait until the next morning to eat again. Therefore, it is best to eat the second meal at either 2:00 PM or 3:00 PM. It normally takes only a short time to adjust to new eating times, and there are suggestions for dealing with hunger, cravings, and hypoglycemia in Chapter 8.

Meal Times - It is best to leave three hours between the last meal of the day and bedtime. However, when following the three-meal plan, it will be a little less than three hours between the third meal and bedtime. (This is another reason the two-meal plan is preferred.) Eat only whole grains and/or one of the exception foods described later in this chapter. This is recommended because whole grains digest more quickly than vegetables, seeds, or nuts. This third meal should be the smallest, simplest meal of the day, equalling no more than 10 to 20 percent of the daily dietary intake. (In the Staying Well segment, fruit is also an option for a third meal.)

Schedules - If the 3-C Schedule absolutely will not fit in with employment requirements, it is possible to eat earlier in the morning. Simply arise a little earlier and start the entire schedule earlier. Moving the schedule to later in the day is not recommended, especially when using the three-meal plan because then, in addition to other problems, one would be eating too late in the day.

Water - Drinking the required amounts of water on the 3-C Program may increase the number of times a person urinates during the day; however, there is no need for concern. Eventually, the muscles of the bladder will strengthen and voiding will occur less often, even though larger amounts will be voided each time. Increased water intake late in the evening may interrupt a good night's sleep. Therefore, it would be better to drink all of one's daily water requirement by late afternoon, saving only one glass for the evening. A reminder of water drinking guidelines: No water for 30 minutes before a meal or 60 minutes after a meal. No liquids with meals, with the exception of a digestive drink, which will be discussed later in this chapter. (Any 3-C

Helpers can be either added to the digestive drink or can be swallowed with a bite of food.)

Exercise - "Light activity" immediately before or after meals refers to housework, gardening, shopping, and other normal activities. In order to avoid **delay** in the digestion process, it is best to wait at least two to three hours after eating before performing strenuous exercise or activity, or reclining. (See Chapter 3, Digestion Principles.)

Make certain that any changes made to the schedule are kept to the very minimum and occur only when absolutely necessary. This schedule is a foundation of the 3-C Program, ensuring that all components are utilized in a regular, rhythmical fashion that will promote recovery. Take heart that employing this new schedule will become easier as time goes by. Do not give up simply because it seems too restrictive at first.

Keeping A Journal

Keeping a journal of what was eaten, how a person feels, reactions noted, and amounts of 3-C Helpers is especially helpful in the beginning of this program. A journal is particularly useful in distinguishing die-off from allergic reactions, which may appear anywhere between immediately and 24 hours later. For instance, if someone wakes up feeling bad one day, it is sometimes difficult to know why. Referring to a journal can show what was eaten or amounts of 3-C Helpers taken the previous day that could provoke cleansing, therefore, symptoms. Even though it may seem time-consuming to keep a journal, this effort serves as a valuable tool.

A journal can be kept on a simple yellow tablet in the kitchen; however, some Candida patients find it easier to type the questions to be answered on a blank page, making copies of this sheet and filling one out each day. Either way, the simple requirements of keeping a journal are to record what was eaten, how the person felt, and what 3-C Helpers were taken. After any allergies, die-off, or other symptoms have subsided, there will be no need to keep a journal.

Sample Questions For The Journal

TODAY'S DATE

MORNING ENTRY

HOW DID I FEEL WHEN I WOKE UP THIS MORNING?

WHAT DID I EAT FOR MY FIRST MEAL?

AMOUNT OF 3-C HELPERS TAKEN?

DID I NOTICE ANYTHING UNUSUAL, EITHER IMMEDIATELY AFTER EATING OR SEVERAL HOURS AFTER EATING, SUCH AS FATIGUE, HEADACHE, DEPRESSION, OR ANY OTHER ALLERGIC SYMPTOMS?

HOW CLOSE AM I TO FULFILLING MY 3-C WATER REQUIREMENT?

EVENING ENTRY

WHAT DID I EAT FOR MY SECOND (AND THIRD, IF APPLICABLE) MEAL?

WHAT AMOUNTS OF 3-C HELPERS TAKEN?

DID I NOTICE ANYTHING UNUSUAL, EITHER IMMEDIATELY AFTER EATING OR SEVERAL HOURS AFTER EATING, SUCH AS FATIGUE, HEADACHE, DEPRESSION, OR ANY OTHER ALLERGIC SYMPTOMS?

HAVE I CONSUMED ALL OF MY DAILY WATER REQUIREMENT?

THE 3-C DIET

Once a new schedule has been implemented, understanding what foods can and cannot promote recovery is critical. Many of these foods were discussed in Chapter 3, as well as other chapters, and there are additional sources of recommended reading in the Reference Section.

Although many Candida diets typically exclude certain foods that are perceived to feed yeast, there are other foods that should be temporarily or permanently removed from the diet simply because they do nothing to promote good health and often prevent it.

FOODS TO AVOID

During Getting Well	During Getting Well & Staying Well
All Yeast & Yeast Products	ANYTHING from an Animal
All Mushrooms	Sugar, Artificial Sweeteners
All Fruit	Baking Soda and Powder
All Nuts	Anything Fermented
All Soy	Preservatives, Additives,
All Fats (Solid and Liquid)	and Chemicals

Remember that starting the 3-C Program means avoiding *all* foods listed in both columns. However, following recovery, foods from the first column may be added back into the diet according to the recommendations of Chapter 7, Staying Well. Foods from the second column, of course, should always be either totally avoided or strictly limited, even after one is well. Since some of these foods are prohibited due to being refined or concentrated, it may be helpful to review the concentration theory in Chapter 3.

Below is a more in-depth look at these foods:

—All yeasts, including nutritional food yeast and baker's yeast, are to be strictly avoided, as well as any product containing yeast. Likewise, mushrooms, which are fungi, should be eliminated from the diet.

—Fruits contain sugar. For a healthy individual, these complex carbohydrate sugars are more easily assimilated and gradually released into the bloodstream, thus providing natural energy. However, they can play tremendous havoc with a Candida patient's blood sugar and yeast levels.

—Nuts, although very nourishing, are a concentrated food that is more difficult to digest. In addition, nuts may contain mold.

—Soy products are usually concentrated or refined, making them more difficult to digest, and should be totally eliminated until Staying Well. Even cooked soybeans seem to be a little more difficult for some to digest than other beans (legumes), although they are definitely easier to digest in their natural state than in a refined or concentrated one. For this reason, soybeans are one of the last beans to be included in the diet in Getting Well.

—All fats, whether in solid form (such as lard or vegetable shortening) or liquid form (such as seed and vegetable oils), will be eliminated in Getting Well. This includes *every* single type of free-flowing oil such as safflower, sunflower, corn, olive, etc. While many foods are either refined or concentrated, fats in the form of oils are one of the most damaging due to their extensive use in nearly all packaged food products, as well as in cooking.

Aside from the concentration factor, fats from dietary sources may form free radicals in the body that, combined with excessive sunlight, promote skin cancer. Processed oils are subjected to chemicals and are void of most nutrients. Inside the body, saturated fats tend to adhere to other foods, making everything more difficult to digest, as well as raising cholesterol levels. Their damage often appears on the outside of the body as well since they are a major source of empty calories. The use of spray-type oils is also discouraged since all vegetable sprays may contain soybean products, alcohol, and certain propellants that can cause food sensitivities. Tips for baking without oil appear in the recipe section. After recovery, vegetable oils may be used in small amounts. (See Chapter 7, Staying Well.)

—Animal products (meat) and animal by-products (eggs and dairy) are foods that should be eliminated totally during Getting Well. In fact, if one would like to maintain optimum health for the rest of her or his life, these foods should never be added back into the diet. Animal products are not only connected to disease but are low in fiber and high in cholesterol and saturated fat, which tends to make the outer membranes of cells "thick." Not only can this thickening of the cell promote cancer, but it also makes absorption of nutrients more difficult. Carefully inspect ingredient labels because animal products are often included in other products, such as gelatin.

—Sugar, sugar substitutes, and all sweeteners, including refined sugar, brown sugar, cane sugar, turbinado, molasses, honey, rice syrup, corn syrup, sorghum, barley malt, maple syrup, dextrose, maltose, glucose, sorbitol, mannitol, sucrose, and fructose (fruit sugar) must be eliminated in Getting Well. Many physical and mental disorders, such as alcoholism, hypertension, skin diseases, kidney, and liver problems, have been connected to excessive sugar. Triglyceride levels are elevated by sugar, which contributes to cholesterol in the arteries and causes heart disease. Sugar also interferes with the absorption of certain vitamins and minerals, such as calcium and phosphorus, upsetting the central nervous system and creating deficiencies.

Even a little sugar can be catastrophic for someone with Candida because *Candida albicans* grows rapidly on a sugar medium. Also, since recovery from Candida is dependent on strengthening the immune system, it is important to know that sugar reduces white blood cells, which are the protectors of the immune system. The chart below shows how even small amounts of sugar greatly diminish the effectiveness of white blood cells, thereby weakening the immune system.

EFFECT OF SUGAR INTAKE ON ABILITY
OF WHITE BLOOD CELLS TO DESTROY BACTERIA

Teaspoons Of Sugar Eaten At One Time By Average Adult	Number Of Bacteria Destroyed By Each White Blood Cell	Percentage Decrease In Ability To Destroy Bacteria
0	14	0
6	10	25%
12	6	60%
18	2	85%
24	1	92%
Uncontrolled Diabetic	1	92%

Artificial sweeteners damage the immune system in much the same way that sugar does but also have the added danger of their chemical composition. It will probably be years before the hazardous effects of artificial sweeteners are truly realized; therefore, they should be avoided.

Salt - Since excessive salt in the diet has also been connected with several unhealthy conditions, many people have been lowering their salt intake. However, it could be that what is added to salt or the way in which salt is processed may be responsible for its bad reputation. Normal table salt begins as a saline solution. After processing and kiln drying at temperatures of 350-400 degrees, its natural state is changed and nearly all trace minerals are lost. Then chemicals are added (silico aluminate, tri-calcium phosphate, magnesium carbonate, sodium bicarbonate, and yellow prussiate of soda, just to name a few). These are added to bleach the salt, prevent caking, and so the salt will pour freely, even on rainy days.

Many people are using salt substitutes made of potassium chloride rather than sodium chloride. However, these can cause a dangerous rise of potassium levels in the blood. Unfortunately, once-nutritious sea salt is now a victim of contaminated waters, in addition to processing techniques such as heating and refining, and may have additives, preservatives, or other chemicals added. Fermented products are also not ideal salt substitutes since they typically have a high sodium level as well as other detriments.

Several safe alternatives for processed salt exist. *RealSalt* is made from natural rock salt, which is high in minerals and has never been kiln dried, bleached, or had chemicals added. This salt is simply crushed, screened, and packaged. Another option is to use a seasoning that has a low-sodium level, such as *Vege-Sal or Lush'n'Lemon*, which are all derived from vegetables. Avoid products, such as *Spike*, that contain yeast. However, since allergies are a problem for many Candida patients, it may be wise to avoid complex seasonings at first because they include multiple ingredients that could cause reactions. For those accustomed to using lots of salt in their diet, salt intake should be limited to less than 1/2 teaspoon per day at first and gradually reduced to 1/4 teaspoon.

—Baking soda and baking powder are substances that leave large amounts of salts and/or aluminum in the body and have been associated with many health problems, including Alzheimer's disease. Aside from this devastating illness, these products destroy vitamins in food and inflame and erode the lining of the stomach, contributing to various stomach disorders (including indigestion, ulcers, and stomach cancer) and causing gall bladder problems.

—Spices such as white, red, and black pepper, cinnamon, ginger, cloves, mace, mustard, curry, chili, and cayenne powder can also irritate the stomach and other organs due to their chemical composition. These irritants tend to destroy the mucus layer of the intestinal tract, which allows toxins to enter other areas of the body. As a substitute for spices, there are several mild herbs that are less harmful. A list of these appears in Chapter 9, Recipes, Misc.

—Fermented products, such as vinegar, certain soy products (such as tamari, soy sauce, and miso) and, of course, all alcohol products should be strictly avoided. Keep in mind that fermentation is the result of decayed food that forms bacterial growth. This is specifically what Candida patients already have quite enough of! An added danger of fermented products is that they cause the production of certain acids that are harmful to the stomach and nerves and promote cravings. Much like spices, fermented foods weaken the mucous layer of the intestinal wall. Lemon juice is a healthy alternative to these products and can provide a similar taste.

—Preservatives, additives, and other chemicals must be avoided on the 3-C Program. Without listing these individually (see Chapter 4 for a partial listing of food additives), suffice it to say that it is extremely important to check all labels for the obvious as well as seemingly innocent additives such as modified food starches, lactic acid, carrageenan, gums, monosodium glutamate (MSG), dyes, mono and diglycerides, colorings, and flavorings. Naturally, caffeine should be avoided completely.

Foods Allowed

Even though most foods on grocery store shelves today are nutrient-deficient, it is still possible to purchase whole foods that can rejuvenate and maintain good health. While it is always ideal to eat organic foods, they are not absolutely necessary in order to regain health. Simply purchase the freshest whole foods possible and purchase one of several good brands of vegetable-wash products that can remove chemical residue. A diluted hydrogen peroxide solution listed in Chapter 9 can also be used to clean produce. Try to locate a health food store as a reliable source of food or a co-op group that offers substantial savings through volume purchasing. If one has a problem locating suppliers, contact the address given in the "Resources" section of this book.

The 3-C Diet focuses on beans, whole grains, vegetables, and seeds during Getting Well. After recovery, Staying Well will include fruits, nuts, and limited amounts of oil, soy and yeast products. Nearly all packaged foods are eliminated because they are nutrient-deficient in addition to containing many undesirable additives. Within each food group, topics such as nutritional values, which varieties would be best to start with, and how to incorporate them into the diet will be discussed.

Many Candida diets are based on carbohydrate reduction due to the fact that simple carbohydrates, and to some degree, complex carbohydrates, can encourage yeast growth. While this is true, the 3-C Program implements, rather than avoids, the use of complex carbohydrates in a unique approach to recovery. Complex carbohydrates play a vital role in meeting nutritional requirements necessary to rebuild the immune system. Rather than concentrate on the fact that certain complex carbohydrates may "feed" yeast, the focus is on strengthening the immune system so that it can reduce yeast on its own. However, these complex-carbohydrate foods will be introduced into the diet starting with the lower carbohyrates foods first, in most instances.

Usually, within a few weeks one will be consuming all foods included in the bean, whole grain, vegetable, and seed families. However, one will not be required to count carbohydrates or measure amounts of food. Although there are suggested quantities given, eating until one is comfortably full, but not stuffed, is the best guide.

BEANS (LEGUMES)

Legumes are from the vegetable family and are simply dried beans and peas. In the 3-C Program, any reference to "beans" means legumes. This particular food family has been providing nourishment to mankind for centuries. Unfortunately, those in Western cultures have not recognized the value that beans can have in their diet. Beans are excellent sources of carbohydrates, various B-complex vitamins, minerals, fatty and amino acids, and protein. They are low in fat and calories while their natural bulk aids digestion. Beans can help protect from cancer, heart disease, diabetes, excess cholesterol, and hemorrhoids. They also encourage circulation, control blood pressure, and help to thin the blood. Another extremely important advantage of consuming beans in the 3-C Diet concerns their ability to help *stabilize blood sugar levels.*

When contemplating a vegetarian diet, most people are concerned about a lack of protein. (See Chapter 8, Vegetarian Diet Myths.)

However, beans can quite adequately take the place of a protein source in the diet, without the disease risk. An added benefit is that beans also provide essential trace elements and certain minerals and vitamins that meat does not.

Most Candida patients feel they cannot tolerate beans due to indigestion and flatulence (gas). These conditions are most often caused by two unusual trisaccharide starches in beans, which are not easily broken down by normal intestinal enzymes, hence causing gas. Therefore, all beans consumed in the 3-C Diet will be cooked using a method that more thoroughly breaks down these starches. This is a very important process since it will make the beans quite tolerable, even for those who have long avoided them. (See the recipe section for this cooking process.) It is rare that intestinal gas is still a problem after using this or one of the other suggestions in the recipe section.

Naturally, a diet that includes numerous varieties of beans is best since each type of bean provides nutrients slightly different than another. However, as the chart below suggests, there are certain varieties of beans that seem better tolerated in the beginning of the program, despite their carbohydrate level. This is due to the fact that some beans are naturally harder to digest than others, such as soybeans (some experts feel fava and kidney beans also fall into this category), and also because beans metabolize differently in everyone. Sometimes beans higher in carbohydrates will produce a sugar-like effect in very sensitive Candida patients, resulting in hypoglycemia-like symptoms. Some have experienced this with split peas, limas, and black-eyed peas. On the other hand, lentils seem to be well tolerated at first, even though they are actually higher in carbohydrates. Another example is soybeans; they are very low in carbohydrates yet consistently seem more difficult to digest. In other words, beans sometimes metabolize in the body differently than their carbohydrate content would indicate.

The chart below was designed to introduce beans into the diet starting with those varieties that seem best-tolerated by most Candida patients. If one is tolerating most of the varieties in the "Start With" section, then they may try those varieties in the "Add Later" category. Keep in mind that everyone is different and a little experimentation may be necessary.

Most important to remember is that well-cooked beans, other whole foods, and proper exercise will all help to stabilize blood sugar and enable a person to soon include all types of beans in her (or his) diet. The Bean Glossary below will introduce those unfamiliar with beans to some common (and a few uncommon) varieties of beans and recommended uses. However, one need not limit her (or his) use of beans to those listed below. Beans can be substituted for nearly any traditional meat or side dish.

BEANS (LEGUMES)

TYPE (1 cup)	CALORIES	PROTEIN (G)	CARBO-HYDRATES (G)	CALCIUM (MG)	IRON (MG)
START WITH					
Great Northern	210	14.75	37.32	121	3.77
Lentils	231	17.87	39.87	37	6.59
Black	227	15.24	40.78	47	3.60
Pinto	235	14.04	43.86	82	4.47
Garbanzo (Chickpea)	269	14.54	44.95	80	4.74
Adzuki	294	17.29	56.96	63	4.60
ADD LATER					
Black-Eyed Peas	198	13.21	35.51	42	4.29
Lima	217	14.67	39.26	32	4.50
Kidney	225	15.35	40.37	50	5.20
Split Peas	213	16.35	41.37	26	2.52
Cranberry	240	16.53	43.30	89	3.70
Navy	259	15.83	47.89	128	4.51
Pink	252	15.30	47.17	88	3.89
Soybeans	298	28.63	7.07	175	8.84

Nutrient value for some varieties in the "Bean Glossary" was unavailable.

BEAN GLOSSARY

Adzuki (Aduki) - A small, dark red bean that is native to the Orient. They are easily digestible with a delicate, sweet flavor and light texture. Adzuki beans are good sources of protein, phosphorus, potassium, iron, calcium, Vitamins A and B-complex. Great in soups, as sandwich fillings, a substitute for tomato paste, or ground into flour.

Anasazi - An ancient Native American bean, this red-and-white speckled bean is shaped similar to pinto beans. They have a sweet, full flavor perfect for Mexican dishes.

Black (Turtle) - Commonly used in Oriental, Cuban, Central and South American countries, this small, round, dark bean is excellent in soups, stews, and bean patties. They are high in potassium and phosphorus while also providing calcium, iron, Vitamin A, B-complex and protein.

Black-Eyed Peas - This small, white bean with a black "eye" is traditional fare in the southern U.S., Latin America, and India. It serves well for stuffings, soups, casseroles, and salads. Low in fat, these beans provide Vitamins A, B-complex, and C and contain calcium, magnesium, phosphorus, potassium, iron, and protein.

Cannellini - A traditional Italian and Mediterranean bean, this small, white bean with a slightly granular texture can also be used in almost also any dish.

Chickpeas (Garbanzos) - A staple in the Middle East, South America, and India, this tan, round bean has a hearty, robust flavor that is excellent in nearly any dish, especially hummus, falafel balls, soups, stews, sauces, and ground into a flour. Cited as one of the most nutritious beans, chickpeas are high in calcium, phosphorus, and potassium while also providing iron and vitamins A and B-complex.

Fava - Similar to lima beans, these pale to light brown beans have been eaten, especially in Italy and the Middle East, for centuries. These hearty beans have a slightly tough skin that may be removed before eating. Their versatility includes pureeing into sandwich spreads and popping as one would popcorn, as well as other uses. Fava beans are a good source of protein, calcium, iron, phosphorus, and Vitamins A and B-complex.

Great Northern - These large white beans are a favorite in this country. Their mild taste is appropriate for casseroles, stews, and baked beans. They are a good source of protein, calcium, iron, phosphorus, and potassium.

Kidney - This very popular bean is named after its shape. Very tasty, these red beans are among the most versatile, being used in chili, salads, soups, and stews. High in protein, these beans also provide phosphorus, potassium, iron, calcium, and Vitamins A and B-complex.

Lentil - A small, flat bean that sports many varieties such as red, green, yellow, or brown; Lentils are traditional fare in the Middle East and the Mediterranean. Also very versatile, they can be prepared in soups, stews, gravies, loaves, salads, or sprouted. They provide protein, calcium, phosphorus, potassium, zinc, iron, and Vitamins A and B-complex.

Lima - Sometimes called "butter" beans, lima beans are flat and may be large or small. A favorite of this country as well as Central and South America, lima beans have a buttery flavor that makes them especially good in soups, salads, and casseroles, or mashed and eaten like potatoes. They provide a good source of protein and are high in iron, potassium, and phosphorus, as well as containing B-complex vitamins.

Mung - More familiar in East Asian countries, these tiny green beans are good in soups or casseroles but are especially noted for delicious sprouts. Sprouted mung beans are a powerhouse of nutrients such as vitamins A, C, and B-complex as well as phosphorus, potassium, calcium, and iron. Cooked mung beans have the same nutrient values except for Vitamin C.

Navy - A cousin to the Great Northern, this small white bean is most typically used for baked beans or in soups. It provides protein, B-complex vitamins, calcium, phosphorus, potassium, and iron.

Peas - Although this bean can be eaten fresh, dried peas are a legume typically available in either green or yellow (which is milder) and may be split or whole. Split peas, which have the outer seed coat removed, will cook in a little less time but are slightly less nutritious. Peas are a good source of Vitamin A, provide a fair amount of B-complex vitamins, and are very high in iron, phosphorus, potassium, and calcium.

Pinto - This speckled brown bean is most commonly found in South and Central America and the southwestern U.S. Its uses include Mexican dishes, soups, casseroles, chili and salads. Pinto beans are very high in protein, calcium, phosphorus, potassium, and iron and contain a good amount of B-complex vitamins.

Red - A cousin to kidney and adzuki beans, the red bean is typically used in this country for chili, soups, and baked beans. They are high in protein and are good sources of phosphorus, iron, calcium, and potassium. Red beans also contain Vitamins A and B-complex.

Soybeans - A major source of protein in the Far East, soybeans are also becoming well-know as a protein source in this country. These yellow medium-sized beans are extremely versatile, as they can be eaten cooked, steamed, ground into flour, cracked into grits or sprouted. Soybeans are a little more difficult to digest than most other beans and need to be soaked and cooked thoroughly.

Cooking charts and directions are addressed in the Recipe section under "Beans (Legumes)."

Whole Grains

Grains and grain products have been staple foods in almost every culture for thousands of years. Grain products are almost too numerous to mention, including breads, pastas, breakfast cereals, bagels, pastries, and many others. Unlike fruits and vegetables, whose health benefits are widely recognized, grains are often not given the credit they deserve. Storehouses of B-vitamins, minerals, essential fatty acids, protein, and complex carbohydrates (refer to "Grain Glossary"), grains play a significant part in recovery through the 3-C Program. However, few people realize that grain products available in stores are most generally made from processed grains that are not nearly as nutritious as fresh "whole" grain products.

A whole grain is a seed that has three parts: the bran, or hull, is the tough outer layer; the germ is the "heart," or life-giving part; and the endosperm is the starchy center. Grains are basically prepared in one of three ways: cooked as a cereal, sprouted, or ground into flour and cooked. Sprouted and cooked whole grains provide a natural, excellent source of nutrition yet only account for a small percentage of grain consumption in the U.S. The majority of grain consumed in this country is processed. Processing grain causes it to quickly lose much of its nutritional value. Any time a kernel of grain is opened, whether it is cracked, milled (ground) into flour, or pressed, it begins to oxidize and lose nutrient value. No wonder white flour has often been referred to as a source of "empty calories." The majority of grain in this country is milled into two types of flours:

Enriched all-purpose white flour: The majority of flour consumed in this country is, unfortunately, the most nutrient-deficient. All-purpose white flour is made by removing the bran and germ from whole wheat, which also removes the natural fiber and most of the nutrients. Additionally, the flour is put through a bleaching process. The term "enriched" is misleading in that it convinces the consumer that all the nutrients removed through processing have been added back in. Actually, what is added back in is some iron, niacin and, two B vitamins. How can that stack up against the 13 different nutrients lost in the refining process? (See chart below.)

NUTRIENTS LOST IN THE REFINING PROCESS OF WHOLE WHEAT

	Percent of Loss
Vitamin B_1 (thiamine)	86
Vitamin B_2 (riboflavin)	70
Vitamin B_6 (pyridoxine)	60
Niacin	86
Iron	84
Folic acid	70
Pantothenic acid	54
Biotin	90
Calcium	50
Phosphorus	78
Copper	75
Magnesium	72
Manganese	71

Commercial whole wheat flour: Consumers who are making an effort to choose food wisely are often being misled by commercial whole wheat flour. Even though it is somewhat better than white flour, commercial whole wheat flour also comes up nutritionally deficient. While it contains most of the bran, the wheat germ has been removed. Since the germ is the portion that contains the "heart" or "life-giving" nutrients, it is easy to see that commercial whole wheat flour, while better than white flour, is also not ideal.

Unfortunately, the reason that commercial millers remove the healthy germ and/or bran portion of the whole grain is strictly monetary. When the germ is removed, so are the moisture-ladened oils. Once these oils are removed, products can "keep" on the grocery store shelves for a long time. Another reason is appearance and consistency of the finished product. Most people prefer white flour because it bakes light and white products more familiar to them, rather than dark, "heavier" products. Realizing the loss of fiber due to removing the bran and germ, some bakeries add cellulose or sawdust to the flour. No one relishes the thought of eating sawdust, and it's even more disheartening to know that the bran and germ which are removed from grain are given to animals for feed!

If sufficient whole grains are part of one's diet, essential fatty acids will not be lacking. However, when the oil-containing germ is purposely removed from whole wheat flour, it shortchanges the consumer of essential fatty acids that are vital to good health. On the other hand, for those millers who do leave the oil-containing germ in the flour, it is virtually impossible to prevent oxidation/rancidity unless the flour is refrigerated. Even then, the shelf-life of refrigerated flour is limited, just as with any other fresh food. Therefore, the problem with buying processed flour is two-fold: 1) When the germ and oil are removed, as with the flour most people are presently purchasing, it yields a product that is sadly lacking in nutrition. Even bugs realize there is little worth having in commercial flour; hence, they are seldom spotted in processed flour. 2) If a flour is purchased that had the germ intact at the time of milling, the flour is very likely rancid unless it was constantly refrigerated.

Discussing flour brings to mind a woman in a health food store who was obviously doing her best to "eat healthier." Encountering a bug in a whole-grain bin, she mentioned that she had never found bugs in flour purchased from the grocery store. It was explained to her there is a good chance the grocery store flour had bugs in it also, prior to being ground at the mill. The truth of the matter is that bugs also need nutrition to survive and they don't find an abundance of it in commercial flours. Therefore, bugs will more commonly be found in whole grains. It is better to have the nutrition from the whole grain (even if a few bugs have to be sorted out) than to rely on flour that cannot nourish the body and probably contains ground-up bugs, anyway!

Consequently, if total nutrition is to be obtained from grains, they must either be cooked and eaten whole, sprouted, or milled into fresh flour. Milling at home allows a person to grind a variety of whole grains while being assured of a fresh, nutritionally-complete food, free from processing chemicals, additives, bugs, and debris. Home mills have come a long way in the last several decades. There are now several electric models that are compact, economical and require virtually no maintenance (see Resource section). Grain milled into fresh flour can be kept in the freezer for several months; therefore, milling does not have to be done on a daily basis.

Becoming "Grain-Wise"

There are many different varieties of whole grains. For those who may be unfamiliar with them, a list follows of some of the more common varieties. Most of these are available, or can be requested, from local food co-ops or health food stores. Every few years, new varieties of "specialty" grains seem to either be developed or reappear in popularity. Such was the case several years ago with Quinoa and Amaranth. The only rules of thumb to follow when experimenting with new grains are: 1) In the beginning of the program, try to purchase organic grains so that it will be easier to determine if a reaction is due to an allergy to the grain itself or to chemicals used in the production of that grain. One does not have to continue using organic grains after some progress has been made. Even though they are better, often they are either unavailable or cost-prohibitive. If so, non-organic is fine. 2) Try new grains in small quantities at first to monitor reactions. 3) Seek out the best methods to store and prepare, keeping in mind that all whole grains need to be cooked longer than typical directions advise. Use the chart in the recipe section as a guideline, comparing the size and hardness of any new whole grains to those that are more familiar.

WHOLE GRAIN SHOPPING LIST

Amaranth
Barley
Buckwheat Groats (preferably not grits)
Corn, whole (must be ground into cornmeal) or fresh cornmeal
Millet
Oat Groats (not old-fashioned, quick-cooking, or oatmeal)
Popcorn
Quinoa
Rice (any that is in its natural state, not processed)
Rye
Spelt
Teff
Triticale
Wheat

Listed below is a Grain Glossary with short descriptions of various whole grains, their uses, and general nutritional value. The recommendations for usage may include the whole grain as well as the whole grain flour. For example, buckwheat could be served as a cereal, pancake, or toasted. Naturally, one would use the whole grains to cook cereal or to toast but would first grind the whole grains into flour to prepare pancakes. Do not limit usage of any whole grain to the recommendations. Instead, experiment with various whole grains for a variety of results.

GRAIN GLOSSARY

Amaranth - The leaves are eaten as a vegetable, and the tiny, dark seeds are used as a grain. It has a mild, sweet, nutty flavor that is delicious for baked goods, hot cereals, and sprouting. The gelantinous quality works well in molding or binding other ingredients together. Amaranth is very high in protein and amino acids, lysine, and methionine as well. Although most whole grains cannot boast significant Vitamin C content, amaranth has an abundance of it, plus calcium, Vitamin A, iron, and fiber. Amaranth contains slightly more fat than most whole grains.

Barley - is available in several different forms – pearled, scotch, pot, hulled, and hull-less. All of these are processed with the exception of *hulled*, so be sure to buy only hulled barley, which contains more of the natural nutrients. The next best would be hull-less. Barley has a nice texture and a mild taste which make it ideal for baking, one-dish meals, soups, stews, and sprouting. Processed barley lacks many nutrients; however, hulled barley has only the outer layers of kernel removed and so has preserved the protein, fiber, minerals, niacin, and thiamine.

Buckwheat - is actually the seeds of an herb, typically called groats. Coarsely ground groats are referred to as grits. Especially while recovering, purchase only buckwheat groats to obtain maximum nutrition. They make an excellent cereal or can be toasted for a taste similar to nuts. The nutritional value of buckwheat groats is comparable to wheat, highlighting lysine, B-complex vitamins, calcium, and phosphorus.

Corn - As opposed to sweet corn, which is eaten as a vegetable, there are several varieties of hard, or "field," corn, such as flint corn (Indian corn), popcorn, and blue corn (which has regained popularity due to its higher protein content). Coarsely ground hard corn is called cornmeal but can also be ground into a fine flour. Hard corn, called "dent" corn, can be purchased from co-ops or sometimes graineries. It can be reconstituted and added to soups, or ground into different textures to make all types of baked products. Hard corn is especially good for flat breads and contains a storehouse of nutrients, such as Vitamins A and B-complex, protein, calcium, iron, zinc, magnesium, phosphorus, and potassium.

Millet - Typically referred to as "bird seed," tiny millet seeds are excellent sprouted, added to casseroles, soups and stews, or used in place of rice. Ground millet makes great waffles and bread. Low in gluten, millet should be combined with a high-gluten flour for rising. Millet also has a gelantinous quality which makes it excellent for molding into loaves and binding other ingredients. This easily-digested grain is high in protein and B-complex vitamins while also containing lecithin, calcium, potassium, magnesium, iron, and phosphorus.

Oats - Even though all forms of oats are nutritious, nutrient values can be quite different depending on the degree of processing. The forms listed begin with the least processed. While whole oats provide protein, B-complex vitamins, potassium, phosphorus, iron, calcium, and magnesium, the more processed varieties contain much less of these nutrients.

Oat groats – the whole kernel oat, with only the hull removed

Steel-cut oats – oat groats that have been cut into small pieces

Rolled Oats – including:

> *Old fashioned* – have been heated and pressed flat
> *Quick-cooking* – sliced, heated and pressed flat
> *Instant* – oat groats precooked, dried, and rolled very thin

Quinoa - (pronounced keen-wah) is actually an herb that produces small seeds; it expands considerably when cooked. Quinoa can be used like rice, added to many dishes, and sprouted. It is very high in protein and amino acids such as methinonine, lysine, and cystine, as well as containing B-complex vitamins, Vitamin E, iron, phosphorus, and calcium. Quinoa also contains slightly more fat than most whole grains.

Rice - Available in many different varieties, rice can vary considerably in nutritional value according to the degree of processing. White rice has less protein and half the vitamins and minerals of brown rice. "Instant" varieties are even less nutritious.

Brown - a whole grain with only the hull removed; may be found in short, medium and long-grain varieties. The longer the rice kernel, the fluffier the finished product.

Converted - has been boiled but no parts have been removed.

White - has virtually all nutritious parts removed in additon to containing additives such as talc, chalk, and preservatives.

Basmati Rice - a nutritious long grain variety that has a natural sweet flavor.

Wild Rice - Not a true member of the rice family, wild rice is actually the seed of a grass that grows in water. It can triple in volume when cooked and can also be popped like popcorn. It is high in amino acids (lysine and methionine), protein, B-complex vitamins, magnesium, zinc, phosphorus and potassium.

Rye - A hearty, wholesome grain that is excellent for breads, rye "berries" (the whole kernel) can also be cooked as a cereal or sprouted. Rye flakes are processed much like rolled oatmeal and are less nutritious than whole rye berries. Whole rye is a storehouse of protein, calcium, iron, magnesium, phosphorus, potassium, and B-complex vitamins.

Spelt - Among the original whole grains known to man, spelt was grown in Europe thousands of years ago. It contains more protein, fat, and fiber than wheat and is a good alternative to wheat-free diets.

Teff - This tiny grain common to the Greeks and Ethiopians is a powerhouse of nutrients. Teff is higher in calcium (17 times higher than wheat or barley), copper and zinc than most other grains.

Triticale - A hybrid variety of wheat developed for greater nutrition. A cross between rye and wheat, triticale has less gluten than wheat but can otherwise replace it in most receipes. It has a higher protein and amino acid content than wheat, as well as various minerals and B-complex vitamins.

Wheat - Clearly the most-used grain in this country, wheat is available in three forms:

Spring or Hard Winter - mostly used in breadmaking.

Soft Red Winter - less protein, used in baking other than bread.

Durum - most often used for processed pasta products.

From these three varieties, wheat can take many forms:

Whole-grain berries can be cooked into either a cereal or are available "cracked" (can also be cooked as a cereal).

Cous-cous is a processed portion of wheat that contains mostly starch and is typically used as a cereal or in place of rice.

Bulgur is processed, precooked wheat that is cracked and dried.

Rolled (or flaked) wheat is similiar to oatmeal flakes.

Farina is a very processed product made from just the starchy part of wheat.

Wheat berries can be sprouted and also grown into grass to be juiced. Unprocessed whole wheat is an excellent source of minerals, B-complex vitamins, and protein; however, the more processed the product, the less nutritious.

Grain Sensitivities

Whole grains rich in natural minerals, salts, and flavors are a vital source of nutrition in the 3-C Program. So important is the nutritional value of whole grains that some people who fail to include them in the diet, especially in the initial stages of the 3-C Program, find they do not progress nearly as quickly or as well as those who do. Avoidance of grains is often due to an unfounded fear that consuming grains may "feed" Candida (due to complex carbohydrates) or may be too difficult to digest. Some people may be avoiding grains due to an actual allergy.

Although some Candida treatment programs indicate that the carbohydrate content of grains could possibly encourage Candida, many health professionals are beginning to understand that diets high in complex carbohydrates are vital for nourishing the immune system, enabling it to better protect itself. Any increase of symptoms one may have experienced in the past by increasing grains or beans will be corrected by proper cooking techniques and offset by other principles of the 3-C Program, such as exercise and *Kyolic* liquid garlic.

If, after proper preparation of whole grains, one still experiences a true allergy, simply stay on the beans, vegetables, small amounts of seeds, and the exception foods. Keep "testing" the whole grains every three weeks to see if they are tolerable. Most people find that the more easily-digested whole grains such as rice, oats, buckwheat, amaranth, millet and barley are good to start with. Corn, whole wheat, and rye can be common allergens, so these whole grains should be added into the diet last.

Grain Preparation

Although some foods, such as most vegetables, are more nourishing if they have a shorter cooking time, other foods, such as beans, whole grains, and starchy vegetables, have nutrients that are difficult to assimilate *unless they are thoroughly cooked*. Thorough cooking helps to split or break down the molecules in these foods that the digestive system cannot accomplish on its own. Undercooked beans, whole grains, and starchy vegetables can cause indigestion, gas, or an overall intolerance (allergies) to these foods. Therefore, the recommended cooking times in the 3-C Program will definitely be longer than any other recommendations one may have previously encountered.

Other methods that can aid in grain tolerability are 1) to cook whole grains for 10 minutes, throw off that water (which contains much of the problem starches) and continue cooking with a pot of clean, fresh water; 2) to dextrinize grain; and 3) to sprout grain. All of these methods are described in the recipe section.

It is not necessary to be concerned about nutrient loss when cooking whole grains for long periods of time, because the majority of nutrients are lost in the first ten minutes of cooking. (See cooking chart and directions in the recipe section, Whole Grains).

WHOLE GRAINS

TYPE (1 cup)	CALORIES	PROTEIN (G)	CARBO-HYDRATES (G)	CALCIUM (MG)	IRON (MG)
START WITH					
Popcorn, popped, plain	25	1.00	5.00	1	0.2
Amaranth, cooked	28	2.78	5.43	276	2.98
Oatmeal, cooked	108	4.50	18.90	15	1.19
Bulgur, cooked	152	5.61	33.81	18	1.75
Rice, wild, cooked	166	6.54	34.99	5	0.99
Buckwheat groats, cooked	182	6.69	39.48	14	1.58
Rice, brown					
long-grain, cooked	216	5.04	44.77	20	0.82
medium-grain, cooked	218	4.51	45.84	20	1.03
Millet, cooked	287	8.42	56.80	8	1.51

No cooked nutritional values are available for the whole grains listed below, therefore, nutritional values will be out of proportion.

TYPE (1 cup)	CALORIES	PROTEIN (G)	CARBO-HYDRATES (G)	CALCIUM (MG)	IRON (MG)
Oat groats	607	26.34	103.39	84	7.37
Quinoa	637	22.27	117.13	102	15.73
ADD LATER					
Rye	567	24.95	117.90	56	4.51
Wheat, soft red winter	556	17.39	124.72	46	5.39
Wheat, hard red spring	631	29.56	130.61	48	6.92
Wheat, hard red winter	628	24.20	136.66	56	6.12
Barley, hulled	651	22.97	135.20	61	6.63
Triticale	646	25.05	138.50	72	4.93

VEGETABLES

Vegetables convert energy from the sun into chlorophyll, which is the lifeblood of the plant. Vegetables provide complex carbohydrates that are high in vitamins, minerals, trace elements, and fiber. The carbohydrates in plants are in the form of starch, which is superior to sugar because it takes longer to digest. This provides a slow release of glucose, maintaining the blood sugar level and helping to avoid hypoglycemia. Many people are under the impression that starchy foods are fattening. To the contrary, these low-calorie foods have been keeping Oriental societies slim and trim for hundreds of years. More to blame would be the toppings that are commonly added to rice or potatoes.

Although eventually the 3-C Diet will include all vegetables, those from the "Brassica" family are excellent to start with. This group of vegetables includes broccoli, brussels sprouts, cauliflower, kale, kohlrabi, and cabbage. This amazing food family has been credited with the ability to heal all types of stomach ailments, regulate stomach acid production, protect against heart disease and high blood pressure, lower cholesterol, and regulate blood sugar. These foods even contain cancer-fighting chemicals and have anti-fungal properties to varying degrees; they actually discourage unhealthy microorganisms, including Candida. A few Candida patients have noticed slight die-off symptoms when initiating a diet incorporating many of these foods.

Most people do not associate vegetables with being sweet, however, they do contain varying amounts of sugar in the form of complex carbohydrates. Although not a problem for a healthy person, even small amounts of sugar from certain vegetables can produce symptoms for Candida patients.

It is unlikely that any vegetables from the "Start With" category will cause problems, unless one is allergic to them. Simply avoid those that do, as there are plenty to choose from. If, after several weeks, there are no problems, and some progress in overall health has been made, move into the "Then Try" category. Naturally, the "sweeter" vegetables from the "Add Later" category will be included in the diet last.

Never try more than one new food every few days so that reactions or intolerances can be accurately detected. Do not progress to higher-carbohydrate foods if experiencing any adverse symptoms. If a vegetable cannot be tolerated, the general rule is to wait three weeks and try it again, or try a different vegetable with approximately the same carbohydrate content. It is difficult to determine how long it will take a person to include all vegetable foods in her or his diet. As recovery progresses, allergies will lessen, blood sugar levels will stabilize, and higher carbohydrate, or "sweeter," vegetables can be tolerated.

In every food group, there are those foods that seem to metabolize in the body differently than their carbohydrate content would indicate. For instance, carrots are a medium-carbohydrate food, yet they are not well tolerated until later. On the other hand, potatoes are a high-carbohydrate food, yet many can tolerate them after the first few weeks. For this reason, certain foods may not appear in ascending carbohydrate order and/or be located in another category. Another exception is head lettuce; because it is a little more difficult to digest, it does not appear in the same category as the leafy varieties.

Discussing vegetables naturally brings about the subject of raw versus cooked. Even though raw foods are very nutritious and contain an abundance of enzymes, they also seem very difficult to digest in many individuals who do not have a properly functioning digestive system. In fact, all-raw food diets for extended periods of time can actually result in an uncommon condition known as pellagra, which damages the gastrointestinal and central nervous system. Therefore, at least some cooked foods that include niacin and protein should be included in the diet.

The 3-C Diet will ensure that plenty of nutrients are provided and recommends that, *only at first*, all vegetables be steamed. They should not be "cooked to death" but steamed just until a fork can be easily inserted. Remember, the digestive system needs to be "babied" until it has begun to heal and function properly again. Then, as progress is made, one can begin to include raw vegetables in the diet. Ultimately, the proper balance of vegetables in the 3-C Program is half steamed and half raw.

VEGETABLES

TYPE	AMOUNT	CALORIES	PROTEIN (G)	CARBO-HYDRATES (G)	CALCIUM (MG)	IRON (MG)
START WITH						
Lettuce, Romain	1/2 c	4	0.45	0.66	10	0.31
Chard, Swiss	1/2 c	3	0.32	0.67	9	0.32
Lettuce, Endive	1/2 c	4	0.31	0.84	13	0.21
Spinach	1/2 c	6	0.80	0.98	28	0.76
Garlic	1 clove	4	0.19	0.99	5	0.05
Mustard Greens, cooked*	1/2 c	11	1.58	1.47	52	0.49
Cucumber	1/2 c	7	0.28	.51	7	0.14
Shallots	1 Tbls	7	0.25	1.68	4	0.12
Parsley	1/2 c	10	0.66	2.07	39	1.86
Radishes	1/2 c	10	0.35	2.08	12	0.17
Cabbage	1/2 c	10	0.49	2.14	18	0.17
Celery	1/2 c	9	0.39	2.18	22	0.29
Broccoli	1/2 c	12	1.31	2.31	21	0.39
Cauliflower	1/2 c	12	0.99	2.46	14	0.29
Asparagus	1/2 c	15	2.05	2.47	14	0.45
Collards, cooked*	1/2 c	13	1.05	2.51	74	0.39
Pepper, Sweet	1/2 c	12	0.43	2.66	3	0.63
Squash, summer, Scallop, cooked*	1/2 c	14	0.93	2.97	14	0.29
Turnip Greens, cooked*	1/2 c	15	0.82	3.14	99	0.57
Eggplant, cooked*	1/2 c	13	0.40	3.19	3	0.17
Dandelion Greens, cooked*	1/2 c	17	1.04	3.33	73	0.94
Squash, summer, Zuchinni, cooked*	1/2 c	14	0.57	3.54	12	0.32
Kale	1/2 c	21	1.24	3.66	47	0.59
Leeks	1/4 c	16	0.39	3.68	15	0.55
Okra	1/2 c	19	1.00	3.81	41	0.40
Squash, summer, Crookneck, cooked*	1/2 c	18	0.82	3.88	24	0.32
misc. varieties, cooked*	1/2 c	18	0.82	3.88	24	0.32
Beet Greens, cooked*	1/2 c	20	1.85	3.93	82	1.37
Brussel Sprouts	1/2 c	19	1.49	3.94	18	0.62
Turnips	1/2 c	18	0.59	4.05	20	0.20
Tomato, ripe	one	24	.09	5.34	8	0.59
Kohlrabi	1/2 c	24	.48	5.49	20	0.33
Onions	1/2 c	27	0.94	5.86	20	0.29

THEN ADD

Potato, baked with skin*	one	220	4.65	50.97	20	2.75
Lettuce, Iceberg	1 leaf	3	0.20	0.42	4	0.10
Beans, Snap, cooked*	1/2 c	22	.17	4.89	29	0.79
Squash, winter, Spaghetti,						
baked*	1/2 c	23	0.51	5.04	17	0.26
Rutabago	1/2 c	25	0.84	5.69	33	0.36
Carrots	1/2 c	24	0.56	5.58	15	0.27
Squash, winter,						
misc. varieties baked*	1/2 c	39	0.90	8.92	14	0.33
Squash, winter,						
Butternut, baked*	1/2 c	41	0.92	10.70	42	0.61
Hubbard, baked*	1/2 c	51	2.53	11.03	17	0.48
Peas, cooked*	1/2 c	63	4.22	11.28	19	.15
Beets, cooked*	1/2 c	26	0.90	5.69	9	0.53

ADD LATER

Parsnips	1/2 c	50	0.80	12.05	24	0.39
Squash, winter,						
Acorn, baked*	1/2 c	57	1.14	14.87	45	0.95
Artichoke	1 med	65	3.40	15.28	61	2.10
Yam, baked*	1/2 c	79	.01	18.76	9	0.35
Beans, Lima, cooked*	1/2 c	104	5.79	20.09	27	2.08
Corn, cooked*	1/2 c	89	2.72	20.59	2	0.50
Potato, Sweet,						
baked, with skin*	one	118	1.96	27.66	32	0.52

All nutrient values given are for raw vegetables, unless otherwise noted.

* Note – Tomatoes, cucumbers, peppers, and avocados are technically fruits. (Botanically, a fruit is the part of a flowering plant that contains or consists of one or more seeds.) However, because most people typically refer to tomatoes, cucumbers, and peppers as vegetables, they will be so referred to in the the 3-C Program. Avocados are one of the "Exception Foods" described later in this chapter that are easily digested with either vegetables or fruit. However, because they are concentrated, most Candida patients may not tolerate them well at first, or find they can eat them only in limited quantities.

SEEDS

While Americans tend to consider seeds as an occasional snack food, there are many cultures around the world that consider them a valuable source of nutrients. Typically grown on other plants such as flowers or beans, seeds are high in protein, fat, and calories. They are good sources of minerals and B-complex vitamins, and some provide Vitamins E, A, and D. Purchasing seeds and nuts in their hulls or shells is preferable; this covering actually protects them from spoilage and outside chemicals while maintaining their nutritional value. Modern processing techniques often include the use of chemicals such as gas and/or lye to remove the shell or the shell may be treated with wax, lacquer, bleach, or dyes. Health food stores or co-ops are normally a good source for naturally-hulled seeds that have not been roasted in oil or salted.

Seeds are a concentrated product; however, they seem to digest slightly better than nuts, as long as they are consumed in *limited* quantities. For this reason they are permitted in Getting Well, whereas nuts are not. For some people, even seeds are too concentrated in the beginning of the program, and, in this instance, should be reserved for later. After one month or so on the program, try a small amount of seeds at one meal only. If they are well tolerated on several occasions, they can be included in the diet two or three times a week, using no more than two tablespoons at a time.

The most popular seeds are sunflower, sesame, and pumpkin. Sunflower and sesame seeds make an excellent base for sauces and gravies while sesame seed butter, called tahini, is delicious by itself or mixed with garbanzo beans (hummus) and spread on rice cakes. Pumpkin seeds are natural internal cleansers and antifungals that discourage undesirable organisms.

Most people agree that because of their size it is easy to overeat seeds. This is especially true for seed butters; therefore, care should be taken to limit consumption to recommended quantities. Sprouted seeds, however, can be eaten more freely since sprouting renders them more easily digested. They are also high in chlorophyll.

SEEDS*

TYPE	AMOUNT	CALORIES	PROTEIN (G)	CARBO-HYDRATES (G)	CALCIUM (MG)	IRON (MG)
Pumpkin, dried	1 oz	154	6.97	5.06	12	4.25
Sunflower, dried	1 oz	162	6.47	5.33	33	.92
Safflower, dried	1 oz	147	4.59	9.74	22	——
Sesame, dried,	1 Tbsp	52	1.60	2.11	88	1.31

—— indicate a lack of data
*There is no division of "Start With" and "Add Later" In This Chart

EXCEPTION FOODS

Even though fruit is not permitted in the Getting Well segment of the 3-C Program, pineapple is an exception. Also, two foods that are technically fruits, avocados and ripe olives, are permitted in Getting Well because they seem to digest well with either vegetables or fruit.

Pineapple

Understandably, most people are surprised to learn they can have pineapple in the beginning of the program. For a large majority of Candida patients, the relatively low amount of sugar in pineapple does not seem to present a problem. Perhaps the fact that pineapple contains bromeline, a powerful digestive enzyme, accounts for its tolerance. Pineapple is high in carbohydrates and contains potassium as well as other minerals. Vitamins A, B-complex, and C are also present. Fresh, raw pineapple, which contains 85 percent water, is best. If canned pineapple must be eaten, use the type that has no sugar added to the juice.

Wait a few weeks after beginning the program to try a small amount of fresh pineapple. If it is well-tolerated, wait a few days and eat some more. It can be included in the diet several times a week, however, as with most foods, should not be eaten every single day. For those on the three-meal plan, pineapple and a whole grain, or pineapple alone will make an ideal "light" third meal, keeping with the principle of only fruit and/or whole grains for the third meal. The recipe section contains suggestions for selecting and storing pineapples.

Avocados

Many people have never even tried eating an avocado. Although they may not appear appetizing, a cultivated appetite for avocados can result in a life-long love for this delicious fruit/vegetable. The majority of avocados grown in this country come from either Florida or California and are dark-green to purple-black with rough skin (this variety normally contains more oil) or medium-green with a slightly smoother skin. Many avocados sold in this country are imported from Guatemala, Mexico, or the West Indies. They can vary in size, texture and appearance.

Ounce for ounce, avocados contain more solids than most other vegetables or fruits, even though they are 75 percent water. While they contain 5 to 22 percent fat, the fat is monounsaturated and contains no cholesterol. Avocados contain Vitamins A, B-complex, and C, plus phosphorus, calcium, magnesium, potassium, and iron. They are also a source of protein and fiber.

Avocados are sometimes not well-tolerated in the beginning of the 3-C Program, and may cause a response similar to low blood sugar symptoms. It is best to experiment with a small amount of avocado after approximately one month on the program. If no noticeable increase in symptoms nor low blood sugar symptoms appear, try another small amount later in the week. Continue to gradually build up on the amount of avocado but limit intake to no more than one-half avocado per day, at one meal, a few times a week. The recipe section contains suggestions for selecting, storing, and preparing avocados.

Olives

Black olives are also concentrated but, like pineapple, can actually aid the digestive process. They typically tend to be better tolerated than avocados in the beginning of the program. Try a few with a meal, working up to approximately ten at a meal a couple of times per week. Most people are not aware that commercially canned olives are uniformly dark and plump due to either processing or additives. While it is perfectly fine to use commercially canned olives, it would be preferable to locate a source of olives that have not been processed in these manners. Natural olives that are simply picked and soaked in salt water prior to canning are called "tree-ripened" olives. Ask for them at local health food stores or co-ops.

Below is a nutrition chart for pineapple, avocados and olives.

EXCEPTION FOODS

TYPE	AMOUNT	CALORIES	PROTEIN (G)	CARBO-HYDRATES (G)	CALCIUM (MG)	IRON (MG)
Pineapple	1 c. diced	77	0.60	19.21	11	0.57
Avocado,						
Florida	1 medium	339	4.83	27.09	25	1.21
California	1 medium	306	3.64	11.96	19	2.04
Olives,						
ripe mission	3 sm or 2 lg	15	trace	trace	9	0.1

3-C HELPERS

As a rule, the use of vitamin supplements is not recommended while on the 3-C Program for several reasons. First of all, the most superior form in which a vitamin can benefit the body is through the truly natural form of food. That's why it is so important to eat a healthy diet. When consuming healthy food, a body knows exactly how much of a nutrient to absorb and, if working properly, will simply take what it needs, excreting the excess. When eating a balanced diet, there is no possibility of consuming too much of any nutrient that could be potentially harmful to certain organs. On the other hand, concentrated supplements can pose two problems: first, they are difficult for the body to assimilate and digest, which means they are not efficiently utilized. Second, other organs of the body struggle to process and eliminate the complex compositions.

Since one major goal of the 3-C Program is to lighten the load on the digestive system so that it can aid in rebuilding the immune system, all concentrated supplements should be replaced with food nutrients. The only additional products utilized in this program will be those that specifically facilitate strengthening of the immune system, enabling it to discourage Candida on its own. The few 3-C Helpers listed below are warranted in the beginning of the program for *therapeutic* use in stimulating immune recovery.

There are very few people who cannot tolerate the 3-C Helpers. However, 3-C Helpers that may be poorly tolerated, or possibly too expensive to purchase, may be excluded from an individual's diet. Simply employ as many 3-C Helpers as possible and don't worry about the rest. Recovery can take place with or without 3-C Helpers; however, it will take longer without their aid, particularly the *Kyolic* liquid garlic.

As discussed in the beginning of this chapter, 3-C Helpers may encourage beneficial cleansing processes known as detoxification and/or die-off. If one started to use all of these 3-C Helpers at once, severe die-off could occur. Instead, begin with the *Kyolic* liquid garlic and bulking/fiber agents. After approximately one month, if one feels she or he has moved through the largest portion of die-off, another product may be included to aid in replacing some of the "good" bacteria, *lactobacillus acidophilus* (referred to as "acidophilus"). Acidophilus may also cause die-off reactions; therefore, allow some additional time to build up on it. After moving through the initial buildup of acidophilus, the pH balancer may be added.

There is no set timetable in adding 3-C Helpers into the program, nor are there any set dosages. However, experience has provided guidelines that can assist in tolerability so one's schedule is not interruped during die-off. Keep in mind that many Candida patients do not notice die-off while others only to a small degree, Whatever the case, this process is a sign that healing has begun and should be interpreted as such.

GARLIC

Nearly everyone has heard of the natural healing benefits of garlic. It has been used for everything from cardiovascular illness to fighting infection. Due to numerous studies conducted by prestigious scientists and hospitals, garlic has lost its "old wives' tale" connotation and has moved into the ranks of "tried and true." And the results are impressive. The National Cancer Institute (which undertook a one-year study of garlic) and the Loma Linda University School of Medicine have revealed startling information concerning aged garlic extract and its effect on the immune system and Candida. This information gives hope to those who have experienced no success with conventional treatment. In fact, *The New England Journal Of Medicine* confirms that traditional treatments — especially treatment with the anti-fungal drug nystatin — are often not effective in combatting syndromes caused by Candida.

How Does Garlic Work?

The 3-C Program recommends only one type of garlic – Kyolic Aged Garlic Extract (referred to as *Kyolic* liquid garlic). It is a liquid product that strengthens the immune system by acting as a biological response modifier that stimulates the immune system so that *a body's own defense system can conquer harmful organisms on its own*. The National Cancer Institute found that the sulphur compounds of garlic can enter the body's cells and stimulate immune response, according to Dr. Herbert Pierson, toxicologist in the Institute's division of cancer prevention. Researchers at Loma Linda University found that

Kyolic liquid garlic stimulated production of two kinds of white blood cells that are effective in fighting Candida.

In addition to stimulating the immune system, it is theorized that *Kyolic* liquid garlic can actually discourage Candida. In an experiment headed by Dr. Benjamin Lau at Loma Linda University, mice were injected with live Candida organisms. Tests showed Candida circulating in their bloodstream and accumulating in the kidneys. Researchers treated half of the mice with *Kyolic* liquid garlic and found less than one-eight of the Candida in their bloodstream in 24 hours and absolutely none in 48 hours!

Kyolic liquid garlic stimulates white cell activities to damage the membrane walls of the yeast organism. The white blood cells then kill yeast organisms and enzymatically detoxify resulting substances, which are excreted through the kidneys.

Not All Garlic Is The Same

Controversy abounds concerning various types of garlic. Many people are under the impression that garlic is only beneficial if eaten raw, so that a component called "allicin" is preserved. This is not the case. First, allicin dissipates rapidly once a raw clove is opened and exposed to air. Second, allicin is just one member of the garlic sulphur compound family. There are many other sulphur compounds that act as antioxidants, detoxifiers, probiotics, and free-radical quenchers. Third, the National Cancer Institute and researchers at Loma Linda University have found that excessive amounts of raw garlic can have toxic side effects when used in quantities more than those used to flavor foods.

It is important not to confuse *Kyolic* liquid garlic with other garlic preparations that consist of a small amount of garlic suspended in oil. *Kyolic* liquid garlic contains a very potent compound that acts as a catalyst in the body to stimulate antibodies so that a person can rebuild her or his own immune defenses. Without strengthening the immune system, a person can never conquer yeast or any other illness. One benefit so important for some Candida patients is that *Kyolic* liquid garlic is tolerable for those with environmental or chemical sensitivities. Being grown on organic, uncontaminated soil, the seeds have not been treated with formaldehyde (a carcinogen), nor are herbicides and super phosphate fertilizers (high in cadmium) used in the growing of *Kyolic* garlic. *Kyolic* liquid garlic is not fermented; it is processed via natural, cold aging, which destroys any toxic elements otherwise produced by such high concentrations of raw garlic.

Kyolic liquid garlic is most highly recommended for therapeutic results because it is the most potent form available. It can be purchased with or without empty gelatin capsules. If taking a dose of less than one teaspoon, filling the empty capsules with liquid garlic is fine. (Four empty capsules filled with liquid garlic equal approximately one teaspoon.) However, after building up to doses of more than one teaspoon, it is easier to simply take the liquid garlic with a teaspoon.

Antifungal Action Of Garlic (Die-off)

Many people are familiar with die-off symptoms similar to those caused by the use of the prescription antifungal antibiotic, nystatin. However, whereas nystatin simply reduces yeast cells, *Kyolic* liquid garlic strengthens the immune system so that the immune system can combat yeast cells on its own. An added advantage of *Kyolic* liquid garlic is that it is a natural food product and benefits the body in many other ways. For those who have never experienced die-off, it is a series of symptoms that may appear as yeast cells are destroyed and the residue is thrown into the blood stream for elimination. Some symptoms that could include fatigue, irritability, depression, spaciness, headache, aching joints, and minor nausea. Some may simply notice an increase of original symptoms. Remember, even though not always pleasant, this reaction is a *good* sign because it is evidence that yeast is being reduced!

Keep in mind that even small doses of *Kyolic* liquid garlic immediately begin to strengthen the immune system, which in turn begins to destroy yeast. Therefore, die-off can occur anytime after taking *Kyolic* liquid garlic, within several hours or several days. However, most people do not experience die-off until they have reached more substantial doses. It is impossible to predict at what dose enough yeast will be destroyed to cause noticeable die-off symptoms. Please note that not everyone will experience die-off symptoms. Especially if

Kyolic liquid garlic is initiated in small, gradual doses, most people barely notice unpleasant symptoms and some not at all.

Very few people are actually allergic to garlic, but some confuse an allergic reaction with die-off symptoms. Many who are allergic to raw garlic do very well on *Kyolic* garlic products due to the absence of strong oxidizing compounds. However, if one is truly allergic to garlic, continue with all other components of the program for three to four weeks. Then, since allergies normally regress rapidly on the 3-C Program, try one drop of *Kyolic* liquid garlic and wait 24 hours for a reaction. If it is well-tolerated, build drop by drop to a normal dosage.

Dosages

Dosage requirements will vary according to individual needs, the state of an individual's immune system, how much cleansing must be accomplished, or other factors. It is best to start with one-fourth to one-half teaspoon per day *with a meal. Do not take 3-C Helpers or consume food between meals.* If *Kyolic* liquid garlic is taken at the beginning of a meal, followed by a few bites of food, no aftertaste should remain. Gradually increase the dosage by adding a few extra drops every day. After one has advanced to several teaspoons per day, divide the dosage between the first and second meal. For example, if taking four teaspoons per day, take two teaspoons with the first meal and two teaspoons with the second meal. If following the three-meal plan, do not take any 3-C Helpers with the third meal.

If increasing garlic doses causes die-off severe enough to interfere with completing the daily schedule, *go back to the previous dosage that was tolerable.* If one should encounter severe die-off, take a dose of charcoal for immediate relief. (See Additional 3-C Helps in this chapter.) Record any reactions in the daily journal, wait a week or two, and very gradually increase the dosage again. Although there are no exact dosages for everyone, experience has shown that gradually increasing *Kyolic* liquid garlic to a maximum level of six to eight teaspoons per day produces excellent results. Maintain this dosage for at least two months after all adverse symptoms have subsided. Then reduce the dosage by one teaspoon every month until one has tapered off of the liquid garlic totally. In other words, if a person feels really well at the eight-teaspoon dosage, and remains there for two months, that person could then reduce the dosage to seven teaspoons per day for the next month, then six teaspoons per day for the next month, and so on until the liquid garlic is discontinued, provided they are still symptom-free.

At this point, a person can start a maintenance dose of *Kyolic Formula 102*, an aged powdered garlic capsule with food enzymes. These enzymes help digest fat, protein, carbohydrate and cellulose. (Other products under the *Kyolic* label include garlic tablets and several other powdered capsule formulations that are not necessary in the 3-C Program.)

A good maintenance dose is four to six *Kyolic Formula 102* capsules *every* day for at least the next year. For optimum health, most people remain on a maintenance dose permanently. These capsules can be swallowed with a few bites of food, or opened and mixed in with food as a seasoning.

The Author's Experience With Kyolic Liquid Garlic

"Many Candida patients are curious as to how much *Kyolic* liquid garlic I used and for how long. I started taking eight teaspoons of *Kyolic* liquid garlic *every* day and continued this for four months. Then, I reduced that dosage by one teaspoon every month. For example, after four months on eight teaspoons per day, I reduced my dosage to seven teaspoons per day for the next month, then six teaspoons per day for the next and so on until I no longer took liquid garlic. All together, I took *Kyolic* liquid garlic, at various dosage levels, for a total of 11 months. Throughout this entire time, I also took six *Kyolic Formula 102* capsules per day, however, if one is using *Kyolic* liquid garlic, it is not necessary to also take the *Kyolic Formula 102* capsules.

Although many people want to do exactly as the author did, initiating high doses of liquid garlic can cause too many adverse reactions.

ACIDOPHILUS

Since Candida is a condition that originates from depletion and/or destruction of the natural *Lactobacillus acidophilus* in the intestinal tract, it seems reasonable that recovery can be hastened by the use of an acidophilus supplement to help restore the beneficial bacteria level in the intestinal tract. An excellent product to try is *Kyo-Dophilus*, a hypoallergenic acidophilus that is free of dairy, milk, sodium, sugar, yeast, preservatives, artificial colors and flavors. *Kyo-Dophilus* is the only acidophilus that will attach itself to the intestinal wall, thereby guaranteeing colonization. Other acidophilus products may multiply a few times initially, but then disappear. Since this product is heat stable, it requires no refrigeration, which makes it convenient for traveling. It is available at most health food stores.

Dosages

Even though directions on the *Kyo-Dophilus* package recommend an initial dosage of one capsule, it is best to start with only one-fourth to one-half capsule per day taken with either the first or second meal. Simply open the capsule and sprinkle it in with the last few bites of food (it will not affect the flavor of food); or it can be left in the capsule and swallowed with the last few bites of food. Excess *Kyo-Dophilus* can be stored in a covered container and used later by filling empty capsules (the all-vegetable ones are ideal) or by mixing with food.

If one notices increased intestinal problems, gas, or die-off symptoms, remember that replenishing the digestive tract with good bacteria strengthens the immune system much like the *Kyolic* liquid garlic and may cause a response initially. Experience has shown that *Kyo-Dophilus* is especially effective in this restoration. As with the *Kyolic* liquid garlic, simply reduce the acidophilus dosage until it is more tolerable, wait a week or two, and very gradually increase the dosage. Maintain a level of two capsules per day for two weeks and then gradually decrease the dosage back to one per day, where it is ideal to stay until the Getting Well segment of the program has been completed. Again, everyone's need for acidophilus is different, based on how much bacteria needs to be replaced. Unfortunately, *Kyo-Dophilus* was not available at the time of the author's illness.

Digestive Drinks

As discussed in Chapter 4, there are several reasons why the use of juices is not recommended in the 3-C Program. However, there is one exception to this rule: In the beginning of the program and only for *short-term, therapeutic* use, one of two juices should be used to facilitate regulation of stomach acid and enzyme production. These two are cabbage juice and parsley/pineapple drink. While it is not absolutely necessary to use these juices, they are excellent digestive aids, promoting healing of the stomach and digestive system. The cabbage family, for instance, has been recognized by scientists as beneficial in the treatment of cancer, high blood pressure, heart disease, high cholesterol, high blood sugar, ulcers, and other disorders.

Many people are not aware they have digestion problems, while others are. Either way, a digestive drink should be utilized for one month by all persons in the 3-C Program and slightly longer for others, if necessary. Cabbage juice seems to be slightly more effective than the parsley-pineapple drink. Most people are pleasantly surprised to find that cabbage juice tastes better than it sounds, and some have even wanted to continue drinking it longer than necessary. If someone absolutely can't stand the taste of cabbage juice, which is very unusual, please persevere. Most learn to really enjoy it or at least find it tolerable. If one is allergic to cabbage, or would like a variation, try the parsley/pineapple drink. Instructions on preparing these digestive drinks appear in Chapter 9, Miscellaneous Recipes.

While digestive drinks seem to help in regulating the digestive system, they do not take the place of the other principles of the 3-C Program. It is the implementation of all components of the program that will restore the digestive and immune system. Therefore, one should not be overly concerned if they cannot use the digestive drinks for any reason. If a juicer is not available, do not purchase one since good juicers are expensive and the cost cannot be justified for such a short period of time. (Using juices for any other reason is not recommended in either Getting Well or Staying Well.) Many people find it possible to either rent, borrow, or purchase a used juicer reasonably for the short time one is needed.

Bulking/Fiber Agent

To aid in the beneficial cleansing of the intestinal tract, including either psyllium seeds or flax seeds in the diet is recommended. These seeds assist in the cleansing process by "scrubbing" accumulated deposits from the intestines. One tablespoon of either type in the digestive drink, at the first meal only, is ideal. It is not necessary to add them to any other meal. Stir quickly and swallow immediately. If not using a digestive drink, mix the tablespoon of seed in a *small* amount of water (one or two ounces) or mix into food. Use of these seeds may be discontinued after approximately one to two months.

Ph Balancers

"Something green" is always helpful in rebalancing the PH level of the body. There is an excellent product called *Kyo-Green* that aids in immune-building. It is an organically-grown, natural combination of amino acids, vitamins, minerals, chlorophyll, carotene, and enzymes. These life-sustaining foods are derived from rich Bulgarian chlorella, kelp, wheatgrass, and young barley. And *Kyo-Green* actually tastes good! *Kyo-Green* also has the ability to assist the body in cleansing, so die-off symptoms may occur. Start with one-fourth teaspoon and gradually build up to one teaspoon. Many people like to mix this product, along with physillium seeds, in their digestive drink. If not using a digestive drink, simply sprinkle over food, or if absolutely necessary, it could be mixed with no more than one or two ounces of water.

The daily dose can be taken with the first meal or split between the first and second meal; however, do not take with the third meal if following the three-meal plan. *Kyo-Green* is another product that was not available during the author's recovery. A product called *Pines Wheatgrass* was taken. Both of these products are available at most health food stores.

Additional 3-C Helps

The products mentioned below are not as important as the 3-C Helpers; however, many have found them useful for specific situations that seem to affect some Candida patients. These products include charcoal, *Releaf* (PMS formula), *Yeast-Gard*, and internal cleansers.

Charcoal

Since some Candida patients are allergic to many foods or environmental substances, the use of charcoal may come in handy until these allergies have subsided. Because charcoal is effective in assisting the body in cleansing toxins, it is also useful in die-off. What is charcoal? Quite simply, it is a pure carbon substance that has the ability to attach itself to toxins and guide them out of the body. As particles of charcoal move through the body, their many small chambers and cavities attract and bind unwanted materials such as toxins, poisons, chemicals, drugs, or almost anything considered foreign or toxic to the body. Some people may have seen charcoal in the drug store as an aid for intestinal upset and flatulence. Others who reside in the western or southern part of the country may have seen it in a snake-poisoning kit. Most hospitals use charcoal on an emergency basis in severe cases of poison or drug overdose. For this reason, it is sometimes known as the "universal antidote."

Charcoal can be made from many substances, such as wood, coal, coconut, or black walnut shells. In more recent years, the effectiveness of charcoal has been increased by exposing it to steam at high temperatures. This process is called "activation" and enhances the adsorptive power of charcoal. Activated charcoal has approximately twice the potency of regular charcoal, so it is a better buy. Charcoal is pulverized into very fine particles and is most commonly found in capsules or tablets. The capsules are preferred since the tablets require other materials, such as starch or fillers, to bind them together. For this reason, tablets are not quite as effective as capsules, and it is usually necessary to increase the dosage for effectiveness. Charcoal can also be obtained in bulk powder and in a pre-mixed liquid form, which is especially fast and effective for allergic reactions and die-off.

Uses for charcoal are almost too numerous to mention. In addition to poisoning, charcoal is also a natural antidote against various bacteria, viruses, and germs. It is effective for freshening air and water and removing odors, which is helpful for those who are environmentally sensitive. Charcoal poultices on the skin can be used for insect and snake bites, abrasions, infections, and swelling.

Charcoal is a natural, non-toxic, harmless substance for which no allergic reactions have ever been reported. The only effect a person might notice from charcoal is a decrease in digestive transit time and a darkening of the stool. The only adverse effect would stem from the fact that charcoal's absorbent powers, while excellent in "pulling" something bad out of the body, would also render any life-saving medication useless. Since such medication is a chemical, charcoal would absorb it and pull it out of the body. Charcoal is the *only one of either 3-C Helpers (or additional 3-C Helps) that should be taken between meals.* All others are taken with meals. For more complete uses of charcoal or to locate charcoal suppliers, please refer to the Resource section of this book.

PMS Formula

Many women with Candida suffer almost overwhelming premenstrual problems. In the beginning of this program, some women may notice an increase in blood flow during their menstrual period and possibly an increase in cramping. These symptoms appear to result from the major cleansing the body is experiencing and normally subside after a few months. Eventually, they are replaced with normal, regular periods that are less intense.

The principles that comprise the 3-C Program have been tremendously successful in controlling PMS symptoms. However, in the initial stages of the program, severe cases may need some help. In the past, products created for this purpose were not always successful, even if taken several times a day. However, there is now a product called *Releaf* that works exceptionally well. Although the directions on the package advise taking this product twice a day several days before the onset of the menstrual period, it is also effective if taken at the time of symptoms. More importantly, as little as one or two doses seem to provide relief, and most women do not have to take it again until the next menstrual period! Many are amazed that so little of this all-natural herbal preparation works so well. *Releaf* may be purchased at most health food stores.

Yeast-Gard

For those who have problems with chronic yeast vaginitis, there is a vaginal suppository available called *Yeast-Gard*. This product may be utilized to help control irritating vaginal yeast problems locally until the 3-C Program has had a chance to rebalance the body. *Yeast-Gard* suppositories are an all-natural homeopathic remedy that provide excellent temporary relief of symptoms. Tests done at the Wild Rose Clinic in Calgary, Alberta, Canada, over a five-year period, showed that 80 percent of those tested experienced quick, effective relief from symptoms. As with the PMS formula, it should only be necessary to use this product until the yeast is naturally reduced through the use of this program.

There is also a product called *Femicine* that functions on the same principle as *Yeast-Gard*. Additionally, *Femicine* provides relief for burning, itching, and discharge. Look for both of these products in health food stores.

Internal Cleansers

After reading Chapter 3, many are now familiar with the fact that various types of microorganisms can be transmitted to humans through several different sources. The 3-C Program, by way of a healthy diet, exercise, water, and 3-C Helpers, will discourage all but the most stubborn microorganisms. For this reason, it is not necessary to utilize any additional products for various microorganistic infestation in the beginning of the program. Since the body will be experiencing enough cleansing by way of the 3-C Diet, *Kyolic* liquid garlic, and acidophilus, additional intestinal cleansers could result in very severe die-off. The author used an herb called black walnut shortly after starting her recovery program, which resulted in symptoms such as severe nausea, chest pain, diarrhea, and indigestion. Naturally, these symptoms would make it difficult to continue with the 3-C Schedule.

If, after several months on the program, one feels he or she may still have a stubborn infestation problem and would like to treat it specifically, this can be accomplished through the use of natural remedies. There are several herbs that can be used on a *short-term therapeutic* basis only. A few simple guidelines can help:

—Consult a master herbalist or health professional qualified in herbal studies. Explain the preference for either a single herb or a two-herb product for a microorganistic infestation problem, such as worms or parasites. Even though there are several multi-step programs or products that contain numerous herbs, they may do more harm than good at this point since overwhelming the digestive system with multiple herbs may cause **delay** in the digestion process.

—Keep in mind that most instructions for herb dosages will recommend taking six to nine capsules per day; however, it is always best to start with a very small dosage, such as one capsule, or less, per day. If no symptoms appear, slightly increase the dosage the next day. Continue increasing in this manner until the recommended dosage has been reached then maintain this level for approximately two weeks. If a person encounters die-off symptoms, the dosage may need to be lowered and maintained there for a while, then slowly built back up.

—Herbs are a food substance and should always be taken with meals so that **delay** of the digestive system does not occur.

PRINCIPLES THAT REGULATE THE DIGESTIVE SYSTEM

Chew Food Well
Eat Two Or Three Meals A Day With Nothing Between
Liquids Should Not Be Consumed With Meals
Eliminate Eating In The Evenings
Reduce Number Of Foods At Each Meal
Practice Simple Food Combining
Limit Refined And Concentrated Foods
Utilize Proper Exercise At Proper Times
Control Stress

CHAPTER 6

IMPLEMENTING THE 3-C DIET

Even though all components of the 3-C Program work together to bring about good health, diet plays a valuable role. Since many Candida patients are not accustomed to cooking with beans and whole grains, some tips will be given in this chapter to make following the 3-C Diet simple. In fact, if some preparing is done ahead of time, it should take no longer than 10 to 15 minutes to prepare any meal on the 3-C Diet. The sections in this chapter will include preparing a food selection list, meal and menu planning, cooking ahead, miscellaneous meal suggestions, tools and equipment for the kitchen, and suggestions for eating out.

MEAL ORGANIZATION

Below are three easy steps that will facilitate implementation of the 3-C Diet.

1–Preparing A Food Selection List

Make a list of all foods permitted in the beginning of the 3-C Diet. To do this, simply go back to Chapter 5, Getting Well. Following the guidelines in Chapter 5 as to which foods to start with, complete the Food Selection List. Remember to list only the foods under "Start With," leaving out any foods that are known allergens. As one progresses in the program, additional foods in these food groups may be included in this list.

FOOD SELECTION LIST

BEANS	WHOLE GRAINS	VEGETABLES	SEEDS	EXCEPTION FOODS
_____	_____	_____	_____	_____
_____	_____	_____	_____	_____
_____	_____	_____	_____	_____
_____	_____	_____	_____	
_____	_____	_____	_____	
_____	_____	_____		
_____	_____	_____		
_____	_____	_____		
_____	_____	_____		
_____	_____	_____		
_____	_____	_____		
_____	_____	_____		
_____	_____	_____		
_____	_____	_____		
_____	_____	_____		
		_____		
		_____		
		_____		
		_____		
		_____		
		_____		
		_____		
		_____		
		_____		
		_____		

2–Menu and Meal Planning

Next, complete a menu planner for at least one week, using only foods from the Food Selection List. Menu planning is extremely helpful in that it ensures a wide variety of foods are consumed while taking the guesswork out of meal planning. Not only is one assured of adequate nutrition, but can also accomplish meal preparation in less time. Below is a sample menu planner for both two- and three-meal plans. Instructions for obtaining 8 ½ x 11 size sheets (suitable for copying) of the Food Selection List, Two and Three-Meal Schedules and Two and Three-Meal Menu Planners are given in the Resource section of this book.

MENU PLANNER - Two-Meal Plan

	BEANS	WHOLE GRAINS	FIRST VEGETABLE	SECOND VEGETABLE	SEEDS	EXCEPTION FOODS
SUNDAY						
First Meal	____	____	____	____	____	____
Second Meal	____	____	____	____	____	____
MONDAY						
First Meal	____	____	____	____	____	
Second Meal	____	____	____	____	____	
TUESDAY						
First Meal	____	____	____	____	____	____
Second Meal	____	____	____	____	____	____
WEDNESDAY						
First Meal	____	____	____	____	____	____
Second Meal	____	____	____	____	____	____
THURSDAY						
First Meal	____	____	____	____	____	
Second Meal	____	____	____	____	____	
FRIDAY						
First Meal	____	____	____	____	____	____
Second Meal	____	____	____	____	____	____
SATURDAY						
First Meal	____	____	____	____	____	____
Second Meal	____	____	____	____	____	____

MENU PLANNER - Three-Meal Plan

	BEANS	WHOLE GRAINS	FIRST VEGETABLE	SECOND VEGETABLE	SEEDS	EXECPTION FOODS
SUNDAY						
First Meal	___	___	___	___	___	___
Second Meal	___	___	___	___	___	___
Third Meal	___	___	___	___	___	___
MONDAY						
First Meal	___	___	___	___	___	___
Second Meal	___	___	___	___	___	___
Third Meal	___	___	___	___	___	___
TUESDAY						
First Meal	___	___	___	___	___	___
Second Meal	___	___	___	___	___	___
Third Meal	___	___	___	___	___	___
WEDNESDAY						
First Meal	___	___	___	___	___	___
Second Meal	___	___	___	___	___	___
Third Meal	___	___	___	___	___	___
THURSDAY						
First Meal	___	___	___	___	___	___
Second Meal	___	___	___	___	___	___
Third Meal	___	___	___	___	___	___
FRIDAY						
First Meal	___	___	___	___	___	___
Second Meal	___	___	___	___	___	___
Third Meal	___	___	___	___	___	___
SATURDAY						
First Meal	___	___	___	___	___	___
Second Meal	___	___	___	___	___	___
Third Meal	___	___	___	___	___	___

Meal Planning Guidelines

Some guidelines to follow when planning Getting Well meals are:

—Include one bean selection, one whole grain selection, and two vegetables selections at both the first and second meals. If desired, one of the exception foods can be substituted for a vegetable. Both vegetables should be steamed in the beginning of Getting Well (as discussed in Chapter 5, 3-C Foods, Vegetables). After some degree of recovery has been made, try eating one selection of raw vegetables at the first meal along with a steamed vegetable. Always eat raw foods first at a meal. If it is well tolerated, try another raw vegetable selection the next day and so on. The ultimate goal is to eat one raw vegetable and one steamed vegetable at each meal.

—It is very difficult to determine how much food an individual requires at each meal. Naturally, much of this will relate to factors such as a person's weight and activity level. A good rule of thumb is one cup of beans, one cup of whole grains, and a cup of each vegetable per meal. If this is too much food, adjust accordingly. However, do not let cravings determine how much food is appropriate since cravings are not based on need. Good common sense dictates that it is best to eat until one is comfortably full, but not stuffed. Overeating **delays** digestion. Suggestions for cravings, weight gain or loss, gas, and indigestion appear in Chapter 8, Special Concerns.

—In the beginning of Getting Well, consuming beans or whole grains may not be well-tolerated due to allergies. Remember that other components of the program (such as the *Kyolic* liquid garlic and exercise) will help in lessening, and eventually eliminating allergies as the immune system recovers and yeast colonization is reduced. Simply avoid allergic foods initially, testing them again every few weeks. If experiencing symptoms that one feels is due to beans or whole grains, one can wait a few weeks to include whole grains in the diet; however, the beans should be eaten from the very beginning. Within a few weeks, whole grains should be tolerable.

—Make sure the menu plan includes as many foods from the "Start With" food selection lists as one can possibly tolerate in the beginning (but not those in the "Then Try" or " Add Later" section). Ideally, a diet should consist of a wide variety of beans, whole grains and vegetables. Seeds and exception foods in limited quantities will round out the required nutrients.

—It is recommended that the same foods not be eaten for several days in a row. For instance, if one eats pinto beans and cooked barley for the first meal, these foods should not be eaten again for the second meal. Instead, another selection of beans and whole grains should be prepared for the second meal and the leftover pinto beans and barley saved for a day or two later. Naturally, if one does not have any other food for a particular day, eating the same items twice in one day will not do any harm; however, this practice on a regular basis is not ideal. Intentionally avoiding any food or food group simply because time has not been taken to cook other foods or because a particular food is not a favorite would very much hinder progress since each food provides unique nutrients necessary for recovery.

—There are only two food-combining rules to remember in the 3-C Program: Fruits and vegetables should not be combined at the same meal (this will not concern those in Getting Well) and vegetables should not be eaten at the third meal. If following the three-meal plan, only eat whole grains and/or an exception food at the third meal, limiting the amount to no more than 20 percent of the daily food intake. Among other benefits, a light third meal will ensure more efficient stomach-emptying before retiring.

—In Getting Well, it is important to limit the number of different foods consumed to no more than four items at the first and second meal. If one's condition is severe, three items is even better. A third meal is best limited to one or two items. Limiting the number of foods eaten at each meal serves to greatly lighten the load on the digestion process. An example of a first or second meal might be: a bowl of pinto beans (with as little liquid as possible), steamed broccoli, either steamed or raw cauliflower (depending on one's progress), and waffles.

When eating beans, whole grains, vegetables, and seeds, it is fairly easy to count foods, yet adding ingredients to those foods in the cooking process causes many to wonder if every item need be counted. For example, if one cooks a pot of beans, using garlic and onions for seasoning, it is not necessary to count the garlic and onions as two other items, even though technically they are. This is one area that is flexible, to a point. As a general rule, herbs or foods used as seasonings are generally used in very limited quantities and are not counted as a food, providing the number of seasoning ingredients is not too great.

In other words, a little common sense would tell someone not to get carried away and use ten different items for seasonings. However, if someone would blend sunflower seeds to use as a topping on a baked potato, that topping should be counted as a food. This is especially true in the beginning of the program because sunflowers seeds are concentrated (and probably at least two tablespoons were used).

Progressing through the program, one can be a little more lenient with adding one more food to a meal. For instance, a tortilla filled with a mixture of beans, rice, tomato sauce, and olives is actually five foods. This may not cause a problem for most people if they eat no other foods at that meal. As one progresses through Getting Well, they may occasionally include one or two extra items at a meal. Some recipes in the recipe section will reflect this.

3–Cooking Ahead

In today's busy world, many people do not have the time to cook fresh pots of beans and whole grains every day, unless using a pressure cooker. For this reason, it is recommended not only to plan in advance what one will eat but to do as much cooking ahead as possible. Adequate advance planning and cooking provide a ready supply of the two foods that require the most preparation (beans and whole grains). Since these two foods will replace meat in the previous diet, they become the "mainstay" of the 3-C Diet. Having them prepared ahead and frozen would require only thawing them out the night before and a simple steaming of vegetables to complete a meal.

Following the directions for cooking beans and whole grains in the recipe section, cook several batches of beans and whole grains on the Food Selection List. An ideal method is to reserve a morning or afternoon to cook beans and another morning or afternoon to cook whole grains. If all four burners of the stove are used, along with a crockpot or two, enough beans and whole grains can be cooked to last quite a while. A good time to try this is during the first week of the 3-C Program, while following the 3-C Schedule only. Keep in mind that if two days per month are set aside for cooking and storing these two mainstays of the diet, there will be very little time spent over a hot stove the rest of the month. Of course, these calculations may vary based on the number of people eating, individual appetite, and type of bean or whole grain prepared.

After the cooked beans and whole grains cool, they can be stored in the freezer. Glass containers with tight fitting lids, such as canning jars or empty product jars, are ideal, especially for those who are sensitive to plastic. However, *make sure to leave enough space at the top of the jar, because beans and whole grains expand in the freezer and may break the jars*. If glass jars are not available, plastic containers may be used. Putting the empty plastic containers and lids in the freezer overnight beforehand, plus making sure the food has cooled before filling, will cause less leaching of plastic into food.

Other Meal Suggestions

A little bit of preparation will allow a person following the 3-C Diet to handle most "eating" situations. For example, one can still eat out by calling a restaurant to ensure that dietary limitations can be met. Most restaurants will even take an order over the phone; all one has to do is to give his or her name to the waiter upon arriving. Remember, if selection is limited, most restaurants or hotels can provide a baked potato, steamed vegetables, and a salad. Grain cakes, crackers, and dressings can be taken along. If one cannot avoid eating at a "fast food" restaurant, select one that has a salad bar and baked potato option. The "preparation principle" also holds true if invited to someone's house. Call the hostess or host in advance and explain dietary requirements, or offer to bring food along.

Packing lunches should pose no problem with the help of a thermos and an insulated container. Feeding children with foods from the 3-C Diet can range from easy to difficult depending on their age and previous diet. One way to serve cooked beans, whole grains, and vegetables to children who do not care for them is to puree them in the blender, then add to waffle batter and cook for just a little longer than a regular waffle. Pureed beans, whole grains, and vegetables can also be "hidden" in and used to thicken soups or stews and lentil loaves, for example. It may take a little bit of creativity and perseverance; however, if presented with a positive attitude, children are more adaptable than adults.

Keep in mind that *organization is the key to success* when implementing the 3-C Diet. Faithfully completing menu and meal planning each week will prevent the desire to eat foods that can sabotage progress, as well as ensuring that a proper diet is followed. Do not worry about balancing each meal, but rather balance *by the day and the week.* The body is capable of storing nutrients for an adequate amount of time so that if one is ingesting foods rich in nutrients from a wide variety, adequate nourishment will be available.

For many people, the 3-C Diet is very different from what they have typically been consuming. Foods such as beans, whole grains, vegetables, and seeds, simply prepared, may taste bland at first. However, do not despair. Experience shows that palates adapt to a simpler diet after a few weeks. In fact, a person following a similar diet (who was not actually preparing the food) asked after a few weeks, "Who's the new chef?" When trying anything new or different, a positive attitude and a little patience are necessary. Becoming adept at cooking with whole foods takes some time, but the results are worth it.

KITCHEN ORGANIZATION

Many of the "kitchen tools" mentioned below are ideal for preserving nutrition and convenience. Some items may already be part of one's kitchen or can be easily added. However, if it is not possible to purchase some of the more expensive items, consider borrowing them from someone since quite often a friend or family member may have equipment they simply don't use. Another option is to put an ad in a local or trade paper, requesting exactly what is needed and stating whether one would like to buy, rent, or pay someone else for a service, such as grinding grain. If there is a particular brand-name item required, be specific in the ad. Garage sales and flea markets are another good source for some items.

Grain Mill

A review of Chapter 5, Whole Grains, reinforces the fact that higher nutritional value is available from either cooked whole grains or a product made from freshly-ground, whole-grain flour. Once flour has been milled or ground, it quickly oxidizes, losing vital nutrients. There-fore, it is extremely important that any flour used in the 3-C Program be freshly milled and either used immediately or put in the freezer. The best way to accomplish this is to either purchase or have access to a mill since using whole grain flours should become a way of life.

Make sure the grain mill purchased does not create heat during the milling process since heat can destroy nutrition and enzymes contained in whole grain. The mill should use a low-heat impact process as opposed to grinding, which usually involves the use of stones and higher heat. There are several mills on the market now that are electronic, compact, economical, and virtually maintenance-free. They are worth their weight in gold and can produce everything from coarse cornmeal to pastry flour. Check the Resource section of this book for information.

If one cannot afford a mill, check with a local food co-op or health food store concerning the possibility of renting or borrowing a mill or having someone else do the milling.

Blender or Food Processor

One of the most-used and helpful tools for the 3-C Diet is a good-quality blender. Used for making waffle and pancake batter, blending vegetables, thickening soup, sauces, and gravies — a blender is almost indispensible. If purchasing a blender, look for a heavy-duty, semi-com-mercial model with varying speeds. There are several good brands on the market.

Although not as versatile as a blender, a food processor is a handy piece of equipment for large batches of food that can be made ahead of time and frozen. Often, a food processor will give a different consistency to recipes since less liquid is required than for blending.

Water Distiller

Drinking distilled water on the 3-C Program is very important. It is preferable that one obtain distilled water in glass containers. How-ever, it is difficult to obtain good distilled water in glass containers in most areas of the country. If one's only option is to drink distilled water in plastic containers, and he or she is not chemically-sensitive to the

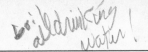

plastic, then the purchased water should be boiled for at least 10 minutes and cooled to room temperature before drinking.

Another reason to boil all purchased distilled water is that the laws regulating distilled water are very lenient and not always adhered to, making it difficult to be sure that one is obtaining truly distilled water. Several random tests around the country showed that plain tap water was being bottled and sold as either spring or distilled water. If having water delivered from a local company, ask them to explain exactly how the distillation system works and if they comply with local or state regulations. Then, contact governing officials to make certain that the water samples are periodically tested for purity. It would even be wise to take a random sample to an independent laboratory for analysis.

In order to have total control of water purity, it is best to either purchase or have access to a water distiller that reaches a proper temperature and also has either a pre- or post-charcoal filter. Unfortunately, some water distiller systems are very expensive, complicated, or don't really do a thorough job. However, there are now several models that are more reasonably priced, compact and convenient. (Refer to the Resource section.)

Cookware/Bakeware

Certain injurious metals, such as aluminum and copper, can be absorbed into the body through cookware. For this reason, it is best to use either good-quality stainless steel or glass pots and pans. (When cooking with glass, reduce oven temperature by 25 degrees.) There are also several brands of non-stick or Teflon-coated cookware and bakeware available, such as Silverstone. Non-stick cookware enables cooking without oils and is ideal for use in the oven or on the range. (Spray-type oils are not recommended since all vegetable sprays may contain soybean products, alcohol, and certain propellants that can cause food sensitivities.) Non-stick cookware and bakeware is best used on low or medium, rather than high heat. Even though non-stick cookware should not "outgas," cooking on lower temperatures will not only help to ensure this, but will also protect the non-stick finish much longer. Simply lengthen cooking time when reducing temperature, which will also reduce nutrient loss.

Juicer

As mentioned in Chapter 5, 3-C Helpers, it is not absolutely necessary to utilize a digestive drink in the beginning of the 3-C Program, but most people find it extremely helpful. If one does not presently own a juicer, consider borrowing or renting one for a short period (such as one or two months). Champion or Acme juicers are excellent quality "press" or "centrifugal" juicers.

Crockpot/Slowcooker

Crockpots are valuable tools for busy people and can be used for cooking beans and whole grains. However, due to the amount of starch in beans, several experts have stated that slightly higher cooking temperatures than provided by some crockpots are necessary to thoroughly break down these starches. A crockpot that reaches a simmer for whole grains and a low boil for beans is adequate. Otherwise, the stovetop method can be used.

Waffle Iron

Most people find that waffles make an excellent bread replacement. They are excellent for sandwiches, travel well, and are versatile. Cooking waffles in a waffle iron without oil may take some practice, but it can be accomplished using an electric temperature-controlled waffle iron with a *Silverstone* or other good quality non-stick coating.

Molds For Making Grain Cakes

Grain cakes are simply cooked grain spooned onto cookie sheets and baked at very low temperatures in the oven. The result is similar to rice cakes. When spooning the grain onto the cookie sheets, it helps to have a mold to provide consistent shape and size. Since there are no molds made specifically for this purpose there are several makeshift items that can be used. A round, open cookie cutter, a canning ring, or the round open cylinder piece of a *Tupperware* hamburger mold (do not use the piece with the handle or the snap cover) will work. If not available, one can simply use a large spoon to smooth and level the grain. Or, hot, cooked grain can be spooned into a meatloaf pan, chilled, then turned out and sliced, and baked. (See recipe section.)

Microwave Ovens And Irradiation

Due to today's hectic lifestyles, cooking with microwaves has become a way of life for many. However, these time-savers may one day be added to a list of "silent killers." While there is no conclusive proof at this time that microwave ovens increase the risk of disease, there is also no concrete proof to show they do not. Microwave ovens that leak nonionizing radiation through the door interlock system may be an increased cancer risk. The Food and Drug Administration has issued a leakage standard of 5 microwatts per square centimeter at 5 cm from the oven surface for the lifetime of ovens manufactured after October 6, 1971. It appears, however, that none of the experts know if this level is really safe. (It is recommended to stay at least two feet away from a microwave oven while it is on.)

Candida patients implementing the 3-C Diet should not cook with microwave ovens, at least during the Getting Well segment of the 3-C Program. Experience has shown several isolated incidents of people who reacted to food that had been microwaved, yet did not when food from the same batches was conventionally cooked. True, these may have been very sensitive individuals, yet it does cause concern, especially for those who may not realize microwave ovens could possibly be a hazard.

Microwave cooking containers are also questionable. According to the Center for Science in the Public Interest, the containers in which food is microwaved, including packaging, plastic wraps, and microwave-safe cookware, may be leaching harmful chemicals into food. Most of these products are unregulated by the government, therefore one has to rely on the manufacturers' claims in assessing their safety. As is quite often the case, the almighty dollar can get in the way of validity.

In 1988, the Food and Drug Administration found that every single package tested out of a group of random products leached chemicals into corn oil within three minutes of microwave cooking. Chemicals can also leach into food through package adhesives (which contain carcinogens), plastic wraps (even those designed specifically for microwave ovens), and plastic containers. If one absolutely must use a microwave in an isolated incidence, make sure to transfer all foods into ceramic or glass containers with lids before heating.

Another potentially-dangerous situation is known as "irradiation." Irradiation is a process used to prolong shelf life, kill insects, and control bacteria by using gamma rays and high-energy electrons. Even though the benefits of irradiation sound wonderful, this process has not been proven safe. In fact, studies to date have shown that even limited amounts of irradiation can raise white cell counts and cause tumors in animals. Naturally, food manufacturers and grocery stores welcome foods with extended shelf-life. Other proponents claim that the small exposure one would receive from an irradiated food is incidental. However, they downplay the fact that it is the sum total of many irradiated foods that needs to be considered. The bottom line is that irradiation is a first cousin to radiation, which is a known danger. Every consumer needs to be very cautious until more studies can determine exactly how irradiation affects health. Be aware that irradiated foods do not have to be labeled "Irradiated." Most often a small, discreet symbol or the word "picowaved" is used, which most consumers either do not see or do not recognize.

PRINCIPLES THAT REGULATE THE DIGESTIVE SYSTEM

Chew Food Well
Eat Two Or Three Meals A Day With Nothing Between
Liquids Should Not Be Consumed With Meals
Eliminate Eating In The Evenings
Reduce Number Of Foods At Each Meal
Practice Simple Food Combining
Limit Refined And Concentrated Foods
Utilize Proper Exercise At Proper Times
Control Stress

CHAPTER 7

STAYING WELL

After successfully completing the Getting Well section of the 3-C Program, some Candida patients are eager to expand food groups or are curious about flexibilities in other areas. On the other hand, many are so thrilled with their new-found health that they hesitate to stray too far from the Getting Well principles. Either way, it is important that one does not try to move into Staying Well before he or she is ready.

Determining when one is ready to move into Staying Well can be tricky, but generally, the patient should be free of all symptoms experienced prior to initiating this program. For instance, is she free of food and environmental allergies? Does she ever experience unexplained fatigue or lethargy? Is she able to work a full day, feeling normally energetic from morning until evening? Only the Candida patient can honestly decide if she (or he) is "symptom-free." If the answer is "no," then it would do no good to think one is ready for the Staying Well segment of the program. In fact, attempting to move into Staying Well too early may sabotage recovery time. For instance, eating fruit on a regular basis before it can be handled well would play havoc with low blood sugar and yeast levels that one has worked so hard to control. Instead, it would be better to continue with the Getting Well segment, giving the body the time it needs to heal.

DIETARY ADDITIONS

If one feels truly ready to move into the Staying Well segment, it is important to introduce new foods into the diet in limited portions and one at a time, waiting at least four or five days before trying a different food. If handled well, amounts and frequency can be increased every few weeks until they are part of one's regular diet. One way to monitor amounts and frequency is when planning the weekly menu. Remember that if eating any of the Staying Well foods cause congestion, fatigue, or a resurgence of prior symptoms, do not continue eating them. Simply wait a little longer and try them again. Below are Staying Well foods, appropriate nutrition charts and approximate guidelines on their usage.

NUTS

Nuts, although very nourishing, are even more concentrated than seeds and are higher in fat and calories. They are slightly more difficult to digest and should be eaten sparingly, especially in the beginning of Staying Well. Nuts can be added into the diet by eating just a few at a meal, once or twice a week. Unfortunately, nuts are so tasty and convenient to eat that it is easy to eat large quantities. However, it is best to gradually build up to no more than two tablespoons of nuts at a meal or the equivalent when using in a recipe. Even healthy people should use no more than two or three tablespoons of nuts at a meal. This recommendation applies permanently. Caution should be used when consuming nut butters since they are also very concentrated. No more than a couple of tablespoons at a one meal per day is recommended. Store nuts in freezer.

NUTS

TYPE	AMOUNT	CALORIES	PROTEIN (G)	CARBO-HYDRATES (G)	CALCIUM (MG)	IRON (MG)
START WITH						
Brazil, dried, unblanched	1 oz	186	4.07	3.64	50	0.97
Macadamia, dried	1 oz	199	2.36	3.90	20	0.68
Pine Nuts, dried	1 oz	146	6.82	4.04	7	2.61
Peanuts, dried	1 oz	161	7.29	4.60	17	0.92
Hazelnuts, dried, unblanched	1 oz	179	3.70	4.35	53	0.93
Hickory, dried	1 oz	187	3.61	5.18	17	0.60
Pecans, dried	1 oz	190	2.20	5.18	10	0.60
Walnuts, dried	1 oz	182	4.06	5.21	27	0.69
Almond, dried, unblanched	1 oz	167	5.66	5.79	75	1.04
Coconut, raw shredded	1/2 c*	142	1.33	6.09	6	0.97
dried, unsweetened	1 oz	187	1.95	6.72	7	0.94
ADD LATER						
Pistachio, dried	1 oz	164	5.84	7.05	38	1.92
Cashews, dry roasted	1 oz	163	4.35	9.29	13	1.70
Acorn, raw	1 oz	105	1.75	11.57	12	0.22

All nuts should be used sparingly

FRUITS

While vegetables are "builders," fruits tend to be "cleansers." Fresh fruits are a wonderful source of energy and carbohydrates. Although low in protein and fiber, they play a different role in the diet due to their abundance of potassium, magnesium, calcium, phosphorus, iron, and vitamins.

Fruit is one of the most difficult foods for Candida patients to add back into the diet. Even though long-awaited and highly-anticipated, too much fruit too soon can cause a return of some symptoms. The author waited approximately one year before trying fruit; however, it is usually not necessary to wait that long. If one is convinced she or he is well, fruit may be introduced into the diet gradually, little by little. Experiencing problems with several "Start With" fruits normally indicates that a little more time is needed before trying fruit.

The majority of fruits are listed according to carbohydrate content, starting with the lowest. First try the fruits under "Start With." (If one has not included pineapple into his or her diet, it is an excellent fruit to begin with.) After the "Start With" fruits have been successfully added back into the diet with no adverse reactions, move to the "Then Add" fruits. Eventually, fruits from "Add Later" can be included.

Just as with vegetables, there are fruits that do not metabolize in the body as their carbohydrate content would indicate. Therefore, some fruits will seem out of "carbohydrate order." For instance, watermelon and peaches are fairly low in carbohydrates, yet seem to metabolize as though they are much sweeter. They, and bananas, should definitely be added into the diet after all other fruit.

FRUIT

TYPE	AMOUNT	CALORIES	PROTEIN (G)	CARBO-HYDRATES (G)	CALCIUM (MG)	IRON (MG)
START WITH						
Pineapple	1 slice	42	0.32	10.41	6	0.31
Apricots	3	51	1.48	11.78	15	0.58
Strawberries	1/2 c	23	0.46	5.24	11	0.29
Lemon	1	17	0.64	5.41	15	0.35
Cranberries	1/2 c	23	0.19	6.02	4	0.10
Blueberries	1/2 c	41	0.49	10.24	5	0.12
Apples	1	81	0.27	21.05	10	0.25
THEN ADD						
Cantaloupe	1/2 c	29	0.70	6.69	9	0.17
Limes	1	20	0.47	7.06	22	0.40
Raspberries	1/2 c	31	0.56	7.12	14	0.35
Honeydew	1/2 c	30	0.38	7.81	5	0.06
Plums	1	36	0.52	8.59	2	0.07
Blackberries	1/2 c	37	0.52	9.19	23	0.41
Tangerines	1	37	0.53	9.40	12	0.09
Cherries, sour, pitted	1/2 c	39	0.78	9.44	12	0.25
Peaches	1	37	0.61	9.65	5	0.10
Grapefruit	half	38	0.75	9.70	14	0.10
Figs	1	37	0.38	9.59	18	0.18
Kiwi	1	46	0.75	11.31	20	0.31
Grapes	1/2 c	48	0.61	12.57	13	1.19
Oranges	1	62	1.23	15.39	52	0.13
Nectarines	1	67	1.28	16.03	6	0.21

ADD LATER

Persimmons	1	93	0.47	24.97	8	0.25
Pears	1	98	0.65	25.09	19	0.41
Papayas	1	117	1.86	29.82	72	0.30
Mangos	1	135	1.06	35.19	21	0.26
Prunes, dried	10	201	2.19	52.70	43	2.08
Raisins	1/2 c	217	2.34	57.37	36	1.51
Watermelon	1/2 c	25	0.50	5.74	6	0.14
Dates	10	228	1.63	61.01	27	0.96
Bananas	1	105	1.18	26.71	7	0.35

* Carbohydrate content of each fruit was not available in consistent proportions.

What Foods To Eat Fruit With

The 3-C Program employs only two simple food-combining rules: Fruits and vegetables should not be eaten at the same meal, and vegetables should not be eaten at the third meal. Up to this point in the program, participants have been employing the latter rule (if they are following the Three-Meal Plan); however, adding fruit back into the diet necessitates compliance with the first rule.

Because fruits and vegetables consist of different chemical compositions that compete with each other for absorption, combining these two food groups can cause gas, indigestion, a decrease in vitamin

SIMPLE FOOD COMBINING

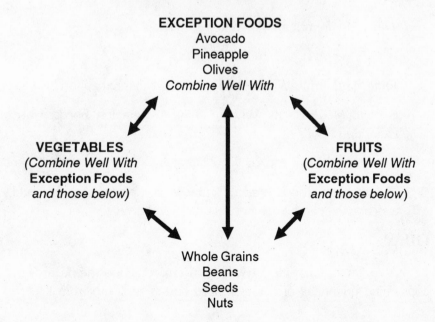

EXCEPTION FOODS
Avocado
Pineapple
Olives
Combine Well With

VEGETABLES
(Combine Well With
Exception Foods
and those below)

FRUITS
(Combine Well With
Exception Foods
and those below)

Whole Grains
Beans
Seeds
Nuts

absorption, and a **delay** in the stomach emptying process. Fruits are much easier to digest than vegetables; therefore, vegetables should not be eaten at the third meal. Very simply put, vegetables can be eaten with any food group except fruit. Likewise, fruit can be eaten with any food group except vegetables.

Since fruit was not included in Getting Well foods, every meal in that segment of the program was more of a dinner/supper type, using beans, whole grains, seeds, and exception foods. Since these are the foods that provide energy and fuel for the day's work, it makes sense to continue eating them early in the day, saving fruit (or even fruit and whole grains) for evening, when less energy is required. Fruit and grains are easier to digest than other food groups. However, if one becomes able to handle fruit well, a fruit meal in place of a vegetable meal as described in "Acceptable" below could be eaten. A list of ideal food groups to choose from at each meal follows:

BEST

First Meal: Beans, Whole Grains, Vegetables, Seeds or Nuts, Exception Foods

Second Meal: Beans, Whole Grains, Vegetables, Seeds or Nuts, Exception Foods

Third Meal: Fruit and/or Whole Grains

ACCEPTABLE

First Meal: Fruit, Whole Grains, Seeds, Nuts, Exception Foods

Second Meal: Beans, Whole Grains, Vegetables, Seeds, Nuts, Exception Foods

Third Meal: Fruit and/or Whole Grains

The exception foods listed in Getting Well — pineapple, olives and avocados — can be eaten with either food group.

OIL

A review of Chapter 3 will help in remembering the hazards of consuming quantities of fat, especially during recovery from illness.

Once recovered, no more than two tablespoons of oil per day (or the equivalent in processed products) is advised. Start with less than this at first and gradually increase the amount. Several good oils to use are unrefined, cold-pressed olive, flaxseed, canola, and safflower. Saturated fat, such as lard and shortening, should always be avoided.

SOY PRODUCTS

Soybeans are a very versatile food. Not only can they be eaten as a cooked bean, sprouted, or ground, they can also be refined into soy products. Although superior to meat, products such as tofu consist of more concentrated amounts of soybeans than the average person could eat in the beans' whole state. Tofu is highly nourishing but should be consumed in very limited quantities when first recovering from illness. Once per week, if tolerated, would be a good starting point. After that, no more than two to three times per week is advised. Consuming soy products too soon can produce adverse symptoms, such as congestion, fatigue, or low blood sugar. Many people have to wait nearly a year before adding concentrated soy products into their diet. Fermented soy products should be avoid permanently.

YEAST PRODUCTS

Many Candida patients find they may have to avoid yeast products for some time, while others do not. It is best to wait to include yeast products into the diet until after fruit, nuts, and oil have been tolerated. Yeast products should be added into the diet gradually, watching closely for any adverse reactions.

Baking yeast is activated by other ingredients during the cooking/baking process. Once baking is complete, the yeast activity decreases, becoming inactive in approximately 24 to 48 hours. Therefore, if yeast products are eaten after this time period, there will be much less "active" bacteria. This is especially true when first adding yeast back into the diet. An overabundance of yeast products is never advisable. There are many other healthy foods that can be used in place of yeast products.

MISCELLANEOUS FLEXIBILITIES

Number of Daily Meals

Limiting meals to two per day, rather than three, is preferable for several reasons. Two meals allow more rest for the digestive system, provide more energy, and better weight control. There appears to be less illness in those who eat only two meals a day with no snacking between. If, however, one wants to resume eating a third meal, remember to eat no later than 6:00 PM, consuming only fruit and/or whole grains, and keeping the intake to no more than 10 to 20 percent of the daily amount. "Breakfast like a king, lunch like a prince, and supper like a pauper" really does provide superior health benefits.

Number Of Items At Each Meal

A review of digestion principles in Chapter 3 substantiates that too many foods at a meal complicate digestion. Therefore, except for special occasions, it is preferable to limit the number of foods at each meal to five, even after recovery.

Exercise

Chapter 4 provides a list of some of the benefits of exercise, but by now most people will have discovered these benefits for themselves. Exercising at the times designated in the 3-C Schedule is the most beneficial, not only during recovery but also for Staying Well. Exercising early in the morning aids in the production of desirable hormones throughout the day, as well as raising energy and metabolism, thereby burning calories at a faster rate for the next six to eight hours.

For those who cannot continue to exercise in the morning, an alternate exercise time can be chosen. If it is impossible to exercise for a full 60 minutes, at least exercise for 30 or 40 minutes continuously. If it is impossible to exercise every day, then a 60-minute routine three or four times a week is best. Whatever time is chosen, the body will benefit even more when exercise is completed regularly.

Keep in mind that exercise played a very significant role in recovery and that discontinuing it too soon could result in negative consequences, such as a return of certain symptoms. If this should happen, one should resume exercise immediately and continue to include it in the daily routine for at least several more months, preferably forever.

STAYING WELL FOREVER

The three golden rules to remember for Staying Well are:

1—If original symptoms return, go back to Getting Well, at least until the problems are rectified. Getting Well is a therapeutic program that heals by rebalancing the body.

2—Staying Well forever is best achieved by sticking as close to Getting Well as possible but using common sense when occasionally indulging in negative lifestyle habits.

3—The immune system takes many, many months to truly rebuild, even though one feels well before then. It is important to give the body time to recover, then always treat it with healthy respect, kindness, and regularity.

PRINCIPLES THAT REGULATE THE DIGESTIVE SYSTEM

Chew Food Well
Eat Two Or Three Meals A Day With Nothing Between
Liquids Should Not Be Consumed With Meals
Eliminate Eating In The Evenings
Reduce Number Of Foods At Each Meal
Practice Simple Food Combining
Limit Refined And Concentrated Foods
Utilize Proper Exercise At Proper Times
Control Stress

CHAPTER 8

SPECIAL CONCERNS

In this chapter, special concerns will be addressed that some may have regarding vegetarianism and meeting nutritional needs. Common concerns regarding adequate protein, calcium, Vitamin D, iron, and Vitamin B_{12} in the diet will be discussed, and food sources will be given. Food charts containing a breakdown of some more debatable nutrients will show that the 3-C Diet can fulfill all nutritional dietary needs, as well as help to protect from degenerative disease. One word of caution: Many new vegetarians seem to fall prey to giving up meat and dairy products only to replace them with junk (nutrient deficient) food. By no standards would this be a healthy diet, and that fact perhaps explains the image held by many of "undernourished" vegetarians.

Besides vegetarian myths, certain conditions common to Candida patients will be discussed, including hypoglycemia, PMS, allergies, medications, cravings, weight loss and gain, flatulence, and indigestion, plus other conditions such as menopause and osteoporosis. It is not the intention to give complete technical background information on these conditions. Instead, the impact that lifestyle choices can have in either eliminating or coping with these conditions will be examined.

VEGETARIAN DIET MYTHS

Protein

The oldest dietary concern in America is protein deficiency. But who decided how much was enough? Surprisingly, it was not an American, but two German scientists in the 19th century who made a discovery and an *assumption* that affects the protein issue even today. The discovery was a method by which plant and animal protein could be measured. The assumption was first that all muscles are largely made up of protein and second that since big, strong German laborers were consuming approximately 118 grams of protein per day, everyone needed at least this amount. Enter the daily minimum requirement, which became internationally accepted and has since been "in the ring" more times than all of history's boxers combined.

Research shows that the body's need for protein is at its highest from ages one to four and again at twelve to sixteen. However, after twenty years of age only enough protein for maintenance is required, except in cases of injury or repair of damaged tissues. So why does the typical American diet provide more than 100 grams of protein per day, even for adults? This excess is partly due to availability and partly due to a tremendous job of marketing by those industries dependent on the sale of high-protein products. Additionally, many health professionals have been sold a bill of goods as to the necessity and benefits of abundant protein diets.

Even the Nutritional Board of the National Research Council of the United States only recommends 56 grams of protein per day for men and 44 grams for women. Likewise, the World Health Organization of the United Nations advocates only 50 grams of protein per day, stating that *even this recommendation provides a large margin of excess.*

Is there a problem with consuming too much protein? Absolutely! Not only is it not required but excess consumption is now being linked to many degenerative diseases. Dr. Barry Brenner from Harvard University says there is a definite correlation between a high-protein diet and kidney disease. That's because a high-protein diet is taxing to the kidneys as well as the liver. Simply put, high-protein foods are hard

177

to digest and assimilate. Excess protein also breaks down tissue and promotes arthritis, cancer, and a host of other diseases. In addition, too much protein also adversely affects calcium absorption (which will be the next topic of discussion in this chapter).

There is no need to fear a protein deficiency while on the 3-C Diet. Protein requirements can easily be met by eating any number of non-animal foods *because virtually every plant food contains protein,* to some degree. Many strict vegetarian choices, such as beans and soy products, are very rich in amino acids. The chart below shows that if a person receives one-third of his or her calories from fruits, one-third from grains or potatoes, and one-third from legumes or greens, the result would be a diet with 13 percent of the calories as protein. This exceeds the published Recommended Dietary Allowance, which is nearly double the amount scientists consider the absolute minimum need. Faced with this data, the only way a strict vegetarian could become protein-deficient would be to simply not consume enough calories to maintain normal weight, to include in their diet only highly-refined foods, or to consume the same few foods exclusively. Yes, strict vegetarians do normally consume less protein than meat eaters or lacto-ovo vegetarians (those who use eggs and dairy products); however, they still obtain abundant protein supplies.

PROTEIN CONTENT OF FOOD GROUPS AS A PERCENTAGE OF CALORIES

Fruits	3.7	Milk, Whole	22.0
Potatoes	6.7	Milk, skim, dry	42.7
Rice	7.1	Eggs, fresh	33.3
Corn	10.0	Cheese, hard	42.6
Wheat flour	13.0	Salmon, canned	49.9
Dry Beans, Peas	22.3	Tuna, canned (low fat)	95.0
Cabbage, fresh	24.4	Chicken	25.5
		Beef	27.4
		Pork	13.9

Many vegetarians and would-be vegetarians hold fast to the myth that it is necessary to eat a combination of foods in order to make a meal "rich enough" in protein. This concept results from the fact that the body is not capable of manufacturing eight out of the 22 amino acids on its own and must therefore rely on the diet to provide these essential amino acids. Since different food groups have different amino-acid strengths and weaknesses, typical protein-complementing theories say it is necessary to balance the amino-acid deficiencies by eating foods from more than one group at each meal to end up with more usable protein. For instance, since beans and whole grains are considered "incomplete proteins," eating each of these foods with another protein source (such as beans with grains or beans with seeds) would be considered a good combination.

While the 3-C Program does advise eating beans and whole grains together, it is not for the purpose of getting enough protein. Rather, this combination, especially in the beginning of the program, tends to help stabilize blood sugar levels, as well as nourish a nutritionally-deficient body. Later on, it is not necessary to eat beans and whole grains at the same meal. Even though the American Dietetic Association still endorses protein complementing, the actual danger lies in the body receiving too much protein.

Food-combining theories differ from protein-complementing theories in that they focus on limiting what foods groups should be eaten together. Compatibility is determined by the types of digestive enzymes needed to digest each food. When the enzymes are not compatible, digestion can run less smoothly, resulting in indigestion and, eventually, disease. While the 3-C Program does endorse a very limited amount of food-combining, it is not as severe as other proponents and consists of two simple guidelines: vegetables and fruits should not be eaten at the same meal, and only fruits and/or whole grains should be eaten at the third meal (if following the three-meal plan).

The 3-C Diet is based on a wide variety of healthy, nutritious foods and supports the theory that eating in this manner will not render the body deficient of any nutrients. It is only necessary to make sure one is eating a wide variety of foods every week from the bean, whole grain, vegetable, and seed family (and, eventually, nuts and fruit) to eliminate the worry of balancing each meal. (Protein content is given for each of these food groups in Chapter 5.) Using a menu planner every week helps to ensure that all dietary needs are being met. (See Chapter 6, Meal Organization.)

Calcium

It is hard to believe that anything could surpass the concern of protein deficiencies; however, something has — calcium! The fear of calcium deficiency is so prevalent today that it has become a common topic not only in offices of health professionals, but at health food stores, grocery stores, bridge clubs, and beauty salons.

Not so long ago, it seemed that only women of the post-menopausal age were concerned about calcium deficiencies. Now it is common to hear that *everyone is at risk* and that osteoporosis, which is a thinning of the bones, is at an all-time high. Once again, industries dependent on the sale of certain calcium-containing products have done a wonderful job of promoting calcium-deficiency campaigns via television commercials, magazine ads, billboards, and brochures. Unfortunately, many health professionals are jumping on the bandwagon.

Due to well-orchestrated advertising by the American Dairy Council, most people are convinced that milk is the perfect solution to the problem of calcium deficiencies and to ensure overall good health. Meanwhile, manufacturers of calcium supplements are reaping the benefits of all this calcium hype. And to further confuse the issue, these supplements are offered in so many various forms, with each manufacturer touting his brand as the "most efficient, best absorbed," that most people don't know which way to turn. Even orange juice and antacids are available with added calcium!

According to independent medical research, as well as various manufacturers of calcium supplements, two facts exist: 1) many people today *are* calcium-deficient, and 2) at the same time, *dairy products and calcium supplements are being consumed more now than ever.* Rather than a true lack of calcium, perhaps the answer to this mystery is that calcium deficiencies are problems of absorption and certain dietary factors that can actually cause people to "lose" calcium from their bodies:

—While dairy products are known for their calcium content, most people do not realize they are probably absorbing very little of it.

Research shows that even if babies have no trouble absorbing calcium from milk, as they grow into adults they are no longer able to efficiently produce the two enzymes, renin and lactase, that are necessary to best absorb calcium from dairy products. Obviously, mother's milk contains the perfect combination of nutritional components necessary to support the growth of a baby during its most rapid time of physical development. Therefore, most people would assume that mother's milk contains even more calcium than cow's milk. However, the opposite is true. Mother's milk contains 80 mg of calcium per cup while cow's milk contains 288 mg per cup. Obviously, baby calves need 288 mg of calcium per cup for *their* growth, but human babies don't need that much.

—Aside from milk, there are other animal foods that affect calcium levels in the body. High protein foods, such as meat, eggs and cheese actually cause the body to "lose calcium". Excess protein is broken down in the liver and excreted via the kidneys in the form of urea. Urea causes the kidneys to work excessively hard by either excreting more calcium, or calcium can remain in the kidneys, forming unwanted deposits.

Other factors that encourage a loss of calcium may be surprising: Caffeine (in coffee, tea, cigarettes or any other form), alcohol, aluminum-containing antacids, diuretics, antibiotics, steroids, too much salt, and phosphates (commonly contained in a large number of processed foods).

Can Lifestyle Affect Calcium Levels?

Many populations that consume lower-than-recommended intakes of calcium do so apparently without ill effects. Could it be they are more physically active than Americans? Dr. A.R. Walker of the South African Institute for Medical Research feels that all of the answers to the calcium controversy will never be had unless a study involving physically fit versus physically unfit is conducted. Research shows that regular, *weight-bearing* exercise can help prevent calcium loss. A good example of this is the consistent results observed from astronauts. The weightless environment of space leads to rapid and profound loss of skeletal mass, despite vigorous physical activity and calcium supplements. All indications show that exercise may be the number one defense against calcium loss.

Even stress predisposes the body to lose calcium! Additionally, since calcium absorption is partly controlled by the intestine, it is important to know that too many varieties of food in the intestine at one time may render calcium unusable. On the other hand, plenty of Vitamin D from sunshine aids the intestine in metabolizing calcium.

—The human body has the ability to absorb the amount of calcium it needs, provided it is given a wholesome diet. For example, a group of boys were fed a high-calcium diet for approximately two months. Then, they and another group of boys were put on an average-calcium diet for the same period of time. The group of boys who had not previously been on a high-calcium diet absorbed an average of 374 mg. of calcium per day from the diet. Yet, the group that had previously been on the high-calcium diet retained only 103 mg. of calcium per day. Therefore, too much calcium in the diet simply isn't necessary. Given a well-rounded diet, the body will better utilize exactly what it needs.

—Calcium supplementation is not the answer since increasing calcium intake does nothing to contribute to laying down of bone, to maintaining the skeleton, or to mending broken bones. However, excess calcium can cause calcium crystals to be deposited in soft tissues throughout the body, eventually incapacitating vital organs and arteries such as the heart, joints, skin, muscles, kidneys, and gallbladder.

In summary, a low-protein diet with an abundance of fresh fruit and vegetables, plenty of weight-bearing exercise, and simplicity at mealtimes can guard against what seems to be a monumental health concern in this country. A glance at the calcium levels of the various food groups in the 3-C Diet, plus the chart, will assure one of receiving an adequate calcium intake.

CALCIUM IN ONE-CUP PORTIONS OF FOODS

Food   *Calcium per cup in Mg.*

Food	Calcium per cup in Mg.
Sesame seed, whole	2064*
Collard greens, cooked	357
Almonds, chopped	304*
Mustard greens, cooked	278
Spinach, cooked	232
Kale, cooked	224
Sunflower seeds	216*
Oatmeal cereal, cooked	191
Cream of wheat, cooked	185
Dandelion greens, cooked	147
Soybeans, cooked	146
Beet greens, cooked	144
Broccoli, cooked	136
Dates, chopped	105*
Beans, cooked	90
Raisins	90*
Dried Apricots	87
Cabbage, cooked	64
Lima beans, cooked	55
Cashew nuts	53*
Prunes	51
Lentils, cooked	50
Brussels sprouts	50
Green snap beans	49
Celery	47
Carrots	41
Green peas	30
Cauliflower	29

* One-cup portions are not practical for these foods and are listed here for comparison only.

Vitamin D

Rickets is a disease that most people associate with a lack of Vitamin D. Even though rickets is no longer a common problem, deficiencies of it may be. Surprisingly, recent studies reveal that Vitamin D is actually more of a hormone than a vitamin. In other words, it is a chemical agent which is synthesized by the skin, carried to the blood or other part of the body, and then affects certain tissues and organs much like a hormone would. Vitamin D plays a crucial part in the calcium/osteoporosis issue. Without Vitamin D, absorption of calcium and phosphorus is greatly impaired, which in turn affects the bones. Also, since most people do not consume calcium and phosphorus in ideal equal proportions, Vitamin D tends to take over for the phosphorus to ensure that the calcium is absorbed.

Any vitamin absolutely necessary for life can be found in plant foods, which were the *original* foods provided by our Creator. Ironically, Vitamin D is almost totally absent in vegetable foods. So where does it come from? In today's typical diet, it occurs in high-fat animal foods such as egg yolk, butter, fat, fatty fishes, and liver; however, *Vitamin D content can vary, depending on how much Vitamin D was in the animal being consumed.* In other words, if one consumes meat from cows that are not exposed to much sunlight, then their flesh will not likely contain much Vitamin D. In fact, consuming as much as one pint of unenriched milk, three tablespoons of butter, and one egg *per day would only provide 65 of the 400 IU recommended per day.*

Because of these inconsistencies in obtaining Vitamin D from animal sources and since it is recommended that the average person obtain 400 IU of Vitamin D per day, adding synthetic Vitamin D has become a common practice. Found in animal feed, milk, breakfast cereals, baby food, imitation dairy products, prepared sauces and mixes, beverages and nearly all flour products, it is not unusual for a person to be consuming 2400 IU of Vitamin D per day! Can too much of this vitamin be toxic? Absolutely! More importantly, this "hormone-vitamin's" long-term use has been associated with coronary disease (since too much vitamin D can cause a loss of magnesium in the heart), high cholesterol, and other degenerative disease, such as arthritis.

Not until man started to "enrich" dairy products with synthetic Vitamin D could dairy products adequately meet the daily minimum requirement. Realizing that first, vegetables are not a good source of Vitamin D and second, that dairy products do not naturally contain adequate Vitamin D, from where did God intend for people to obtain this vital element? Perhaps it was never intended that food be a source of Vitamin D. Research is now showing there is only one completely safe source of Vitamin D — the sun!

A study of veterans who lived in the Chelsea, Massachusetts, Soldiers' Home was done to determine if sunlight is superior to dietary Vitamin D. The entire pilot group remained inside during the winter months and received a minimum of 200 IU of Vitamin D from dairy products, however, one-half were also subjected to full-spectrum lighting to obtain ultraviolet light. The study concluded that those receiving the extra ultraviolet light increased their calcium absorption by 15 percent while those not receiving extra light decreased their absorption by 25 percent. Clearly, the ultraviolet light was more effective than the synthetic Vitamin D found in foods.

How much sunlight is required to maintain a healthy dose of Vitamin D? Not as much as one would think. As little as 15 minutes a day (or even a few minutes for a child) can protect from a Vitamin D deficiency. The body also has the ability to "store" Vitamin D from repeated exposure in warm months to draw on through the winter months when people tend to stay indoors. Ideally, one should try to get out in the fresh air and sunshine for at least a few minutes every day. Then, when convenient, it is advantageous to spend longer periods of time outside such as in exercise, working or just relaxing. Full spectrum lighting inside will also help protect against deficiencies. (See Chapter 4, Sunlight.)

Iron

Although the number of iron-deficient anemics have decreased in the last several decades, iron is still the most widely-deficient nutrient in this country. Assuming that iron from beans, whole grains, and vegetable sources is a poor substitute for the "real" iron found in meat, many health professionals typically feel that vegetarians are more susceptible to iron deficiencies. However, researchers around the world find that vegetarians are not lacking in iron and often consume higher levels of iron than nonvegetarians. Vegetarians also may tend to better absorb iron since iron absorption, like calcium absorption, is affected by other foods in the diet.

Some experts say iron-rich foods must be consumed along with foods that contain Vitamin C. This is not difficult to accomplish in the 3-C Program since many vegetables contain Vitamin C. Also, it may not be necessary to eat Vitamin C foods every single time iron foods are eaten. Another theory deals with the fact that fiber may block the absorption of iron. However, a study conducted by the University of Kansas Medical Center concluded that not every type of fiber depleted iron absorption and that "fiber is not a major determinant of food iron availability."

Just as with calcium, the body knows when it has enough iron and absorbs less from food. Conversely, when there is not enough iron in the body, absorption from food becomes more efficient. Even though the body does have a defense against iron shortages, an increased usage of dairy products containing calcium and phosphorus that bind with iron tend to interfere with the absorption of iron. Instead, including foods in the diet that are high in iron (and Vitamin C) will insure that the body is receiving the amount it needs. Even cooking with iron utensils can provide a source of iron.

FOODS HIGH IN IRON

FOOD	APPROXIMATE MEASURE	IRON, MG PER SERVING	PER 100 GM.
Almonds	12-15	0.7	4.4
Apricots, dried	5 halves	1.5	4.9
Beans, dried, cooked	1/2 cup	2.1	6.9
Lima, dried, cooked	1/2 cup	2.3	7.5
Beet greens, cooked	1/2 cup	2.4	3.2
Brazil nuts	2 medium	0.5	3.4
Bread, whole wheat	1 slice	0.6	2.2
Cashews	6-8	0.8	5.0
Swiss Chard	1/2 cup	1.9	2.5
Coconut, fresh	1/2 ounce	0.3	2.0
Dried	2 tablespoons	0.5	3.6
Cornmeal, degermed, enriched, cooked	1/2 cup	0.4	2.9
Cress, garden	5-8 sprigs	0.3	2.9
Currants, dried	2 tablespoons	0.8	2.7
Dandelion greens	1/2 cup	2.3	3.1
Dates	3-4	0.6	2.1
Figs, dried	2 small	0.9	3.0

FOODS HIGH IN IRON (Continued)

FOOD	APPROXIMATE MEASURE	IRON, MG PER SERVING	PER 100 GM.
Flour,			
all purpose, enriched . . . . 2 tablespoons		0.4	2.9
whole wheat . . . . 2 tablespoons		0.5	3.3
Hazelnuts 10-12		0.6	4.1
Kale . . . . 3/4 cup		1.7	2.2
Lentils, dry, cooked . . . . 1/2 cup		2.2	7.4
Oatmeal, cooked . . . . 1/2 cup		0.7	4.5
Parsley . . . . 10 small sprigs		0.4	4.3
Peaches, dried . . . . 3 halves		1.9	6.9
Peas, dry, cooked . . . . 1/2 cup		1.4	4.7
Pecans . . . . 12 halves		0.4	2.4
Popcorn, popped . . . . 1 cup		0.4	2.7
Prunes, dried . . . . 4 prunes		1.2	3.9
Raisins, dried . . . . 5 tablespoons		1.7	3.3
Rice, brown, cooked . . . . 1/2 cup		0.3	2.0
Rye, whole meal . . . . 1 tablespoon		0.6	3.7

Vitamin B$_{12}$

Controversy abounds concerning B$_{12}$ deficiencies in vegetarians and nonvegetarians alike. Adding to the concern is the fact that previously-trusted tests for B$_{12}$ deficiency are not always accurate. A blood test is the first step in identifying most B$_{12}$ deficiencies. If warranted, a more elaborate test, the Schilling test, is then performed. However, a researcher at the University of Southern California School of Medicine has discovered that this time-honored test can be misleading. Designed to determine if a person is actually absorbing B$_{12}$ from her or his diet, the Schilling test is administered by a mixture of water and radioactive B$_{12}$, which is tracked through the body. Here's the problem: Failing the test means something is amiss in the stomach or small intestine; however, passing the test gives one a clean bill of health despite the fact that they may still be deficient in B$_{12}$.

Actually, B$_{12}$ deficiency is a rare disorder and the overwhelming majority of cases occur in nonvegetarians! Research by Drs. Calvin and Agatha Thrash of Uchee Pines Institute has shown that true deficiency is not so much caused by a lack of B$_{12}$ in the diet but by one of many other factors such as malabsorption, consuming animal products and refined foods, increased elimination, lack of other nutrients due to poor diet, the use of oral contraceptives, and even high doses of Vitamin C or B_1. The most common cause, malabsorption, can be attributed to one of the following: a lack of hydrochloric acid in the stomach, toxic poisoning, use of alcohol, nicotine, caffeine and other drugs, intestinal parasites, disease, or removal of a portion of the intestine. Better B_{12} absorption can be encouraged by chewing properly, leaving plenty of time between meals and limiting the number of foods at each meal.

Is there reason to be concerned about B_{12} deficiencies when first becoming a strict vegetarian? Not initially, because vegetarians can actually maintain necessary B_{12} levels for three to five years without supplements. Therefore, when initiating the 3-C Program, stored amounts of B_{12} in the body will be quite adequate for some time. Additionally, The Drs. Thrash in *Nutrition For Vegetarians*, say, "While vitamins are not synthesized by the body, some, including vitamins K, B_1, folacin, and B_{12}, are synthesized by bacteria in various parts of the body. All of these are produced by microorganisms that normally inhabit the gastrointestinal tract. Vitamin B_{12} is also produced in the mouth, conjunctival sacs, tonsils, nasopharynx, bronchial tree, sinuses, stomach, and small bowel." Except for unusual situations, these sources can actually supply adequate amounts of Vitamin B_{12} for strict vegetarians.

Contrary to popular belief there are several vegetarian sources of Vitamin B_{12}, as one can see from the chart. While these sources may not be constant, it appears that they occur with sufficient frequency to supply the minute quantities of Vitamin B_{12} that are needed by those who are maintaining a good health program.

NATURAL SOURCES OF B$_{12}$

Alfalfa . . . . Amaranth
Dark leafy green Vegetables . . . . Fruit
Olives . . . . Root Vegetables
Seaweed . . . . Soybeans
Wheat

Surface of all lightly washed, raw vegetables

Microorganisms produced in various parts of the body

Some drinking water

SPECIAL HEALTH CONDITIONS

Hypoglycemia (Low Blood Sugar)

Many Candida patients suffer from hypoglycemia-like symptoms, even though tests may not have confirmed true hypoglycemia. Symptoms can include, but are not limited to mild to severe headaches, cravings, allergies, drowsiness, fatigue, mental confusion, poor concentration, irritability, depression, impatience, shakiness, feeling faint, hyperactivity, and rapid heart beat. Many Candida patients may have experienced all or some of these symptoms, to some degree, for years prior to a diagnosis of Candida.

Many "well" individuals may also experience a certain level of some of these symptoms. For instance, people commonly joke about how difficult it can be to stay awake during the afternoon. Others complain they can make it through the workday, but lack energy in the evenings. Working women may find it a struggle to work all day, then care for their family and home in the evenings.

In today's world, it appears that hypoglycemia-like symptoms are more normal than unusual. Yet, when many are tested to see if this could be their problem, they are told their blood sugar levels are normal. Maybe this is the problem: Because so many people do have a lowered blood sugar, the standard, or "norm," has also been lowered. Therefore, when a person with low blood sugar is compared to others whose levels are also low, that person's blood sugar level would appear normal. In other words, low blood sugar levels are so common today, that true low blood sugar levels are now considered normal. However, there is a difference between "normal" and "ideal."

Why are hypoglycemic symptoms so common? Contrary to what most believe, this condition is rarely a result of disease, but more typically brought on by lifestyle. For instance, look at how just one factor, diet, affects blood sugar: A healthy intake of limited amounts of protein, combined with sufficient vitamins, minerals, and complex carbohydrates releases sugar into the bloodstream at a steady, moderate rate, which keeps energy levels constant throughout the day. However, eating sugar, which is a simple carbohydrate that enters the bloodstream rapidly, will very quickly raise the blood sugar level. Even though this may provide quick energy, the pancreas responds to this overload of simple carbohydrates by producing an *abundance of insulin*, which then causes the blood sugar to *drop very low*. This "roller coaster effect" can be paralleled with mood and energy patterns. Severe hypoglycemic reactions common to so many Candida patients typically result from the small amounts of sugar in fruits and even in some vegetables.

Dietary contributors to hypoglycemia (aside from sugar) are often the same contributors to other illnesses. Diets lacking fiber and complex carbohydrates, yet high in protein, as well as drugs such as caffeine, nicotine, and alcohol, will encourage insulin production.

Even the digestive system and other organs can be affected by low blood sugar. As the blood sugar level lowers, it can cause an irritated digestive tract, which will become congested with blood. The liver, muscles, and brain receive less nourishing blood than normal, substantiating why many hypoglycemic symptoms can be mental, as well as physical. If the brain does not have a steady supply of blood and glucose, many of the symptoms previously mentioned will appear. In severe hypoglycemia, extreme patterns of thinking, compulsions, or thoughts of suicide could develop. Many people complain of unexplainable feelings: tingling on the scalp, pressure inside the head, or feeling as though there is a tight band around the skull.

In addition to a poor diet, other lifestyle choices that promote hypoglycemic symptoms, are lack of exercise, eating at irregular times, eating too often and insufficient water intake. Combined lifestyle choices that promote low blood sugar syndrome produce a constant hardship on the body that develops into a vicious cycle. For example, eating too often is not only taxing to the digestive system but also promotes blood levels to first rise, then drop drastically, which causes a hardship on the pancreas.

Just as abusing a machine eventually results in a breakdown, so do constant abuses on the body eventually take their toll. After years of this hypoglycemic syndrome, the end result may very well be diabetes. That's right, even though diabetes represents a high blood sugar level, this condition typically starts out as a low blood sugar problem. Hypoglycemia, then, is potentially more serious than most realize. If unhealthy lifestyles are continued, not only can diabetes result but the whole body suffers an accelerated aging process that encourages degenerative disease of all types.

The good news is that the same lifestyle choices that alleviate symptoms of Candida are also effective in alleviating hypoglycemic symptoms. Below is a review of 3-C principles that will help to stabilize blood sugar levels:

—Sustained exercise everyday is *absolutely* essential and is especially effective if performed early in the morning.

—A diet high in whole foods such as beans, whole grains, vegetables, and seeds is necessary. Fruit and concentrated or refined foods should be avoided until low blood sugar and yeast problems are under control. The pectin in fruit lowers blood sugar after eating, as well as supporting yeast.

—Plenty of water between meals should take the place of snacking since positively *no* eating between meals should occur.

—A *regular* schedule should be followed every day, particularly for mealtimes, bedtimes and exercise.

Candida patients will find that controlling blood sugar levels using these principles will help alleviate a multitude of symptoms in the beginning of the program, such as allergies and fatigue. Experience has shown that a *lack of exercise,* even for one or two days, may *cause adverse symptoms to reappear very quickly.* This is understandable since proper exercise at proper times not only strengthens the immune system but promotes digestion. When the digestive system is functioning efficiently, food is assimilated better, which discourages allergies.

While improving lifestyle choices will stabilize low blood sugar, the length of time it takes to accomplish this will vary for everyone. Predicting how long it will take an over-worked digestive system, a weakened immune system, and an unregulated pancreas to once again function normally is difficult. However, most people report increased energy within a few weeks. In fact, were it not for the fact that yeast die-off is sometimes noticeable in Candida cases, balancing low blood sugar could be accomplished in a short time by simply changing lifestyles. However long these processes take, one should allow ample time and not become discouraged. Favorable lifestyle choices, combined with regularity in all areas, will provide not only balanced blood sugar levels but a longer, healthier life.

PMS

Nearly 90 percent of all women in their reproductive years experience PMS symptoms. Even though most health professionals realize that PMS is the body's reaction to hormonal changes, they still struggle to explain the cause of this condition and how to treat it. In addressing the problems of Candida patients, it is apparent that a large share of these women also suffer from PMS. Many symptoms of Candida and PMS seem to intertwine, such as weight gain and bloating, digestive problems, acne, cramps, and breast tenderness. Likewise, PMS symptoms can include hypoglycemic symptoms, such as increased appetite, cravings, irritability, tension, mood swings, dizziness, fatigue, and headaches. In other words, PMS, like Candida and hypoglycemia, seems to be a syndrome representing a collection of symptoms that may increase during the highest levels of hormonal changes. Dr. William Crook feels that many women develop PMS because of a hormonal abnormality induced by a deficient immune system associated with Candida.

Many women who followed the 3-C Program due to Candida were surprised to find that symptoms of PMS also disappeared. The key to resolving the PMS dilemma seems to be regularity of lifestyle, *especially in diet and exercise*, as well as adequate water, sunshine, rest, and controlling stress. The elimination of certain aggravating foods and substances listed below will help in alleviating a PMS condition:

FOODS TO AVOID WHEN CORRECTING PMS SYNDROME

Coffee	Alcohol
Tea	Tobacco
Soft drinks	Medications
Animal products	Preservatives
Fats	Spices
Salt	MSG

All refined, fermented, smoked or pickled foods.

Correcting a PMS situation that has probably been "in the works" for many months or years will not occur overnight, although some women do experience improvement from the very beginning. More commonly reported is that the first one to three months of the 3-C Program found them feeling much better physically, *except during their menstrual periods.* During that time, the body seems to do an intense "cleansing" of the female organs that may result in heavier-than-normal bleeding, slightly more cramping and other intensified symptoms. However, this should not be cause for alarm. Eventually, menstrual periods become regular, with minimal or no discomfort. In fact, consistent reports of "This is the first normal menstrual period I have had in years," are very common. Just as with hypoglycemia and Candida, incorporating the regulating principles of the 3-C Program will help to alleviate PMS problems.

Menopause And Estrogen

Menopause literally means "cessation of menses" and refers to that period in a woman's life when reproductive function has come to an end. A woman may also be confronted with menopausal symptoms due to the surgical removal of her ovaries. Either way, there is a decline in hormonal secretion typically referred to as "the change of life." Symptoms of menopause are brought on by an estrogen deficiency that upsets the hypothalamic control of the autonomic nervous system. Hot flashes, sweats, depression, apprehension, nervousness, insomnia, headaches, crawling sensation of the skin, dryness, itching, heart palpitations, and many other symptoms have been associated with menopause for some women. Others seem to breeze through this transition with either no serious problems or symptoms that are short-lived.

Previously, hormonal replacement therapy, such as estrogen or estrogen-progesterone combinations, was thought to be the only way to relieve some of the frustrating symptoms of menopause. However, much controversy concerning long-term safety of these preparations abounds. Women presently taking estrogen owe it to themselves to study the facts. The association of estrogen with certain cancers, such as breast, ovarian, and endometrial, is frightening. Unfortunately, some women taking estrogen are in hopes it will also slow the aging process; however, statistics show that estrogen has no affect on early aging, nor does it reduce the risk of developing osteoporosis.

Will estrogen interfere with the 3-C Program? First of all, taking hormones of any kind poses a serious health risk, including encouragement of yeast colonization, since yeast seems to thrive on hormones. Second, if all principles of the 3-C Program are followed, in addition to recommendations below, estrogen therapy is not necessary.

Exciting news is that there are certain foods that contain plant steroids similar to estrogen. In fact, it was demonstrated that post-menopausal women who were consuming these foods actually started bleeding when they were withdrawn all at one time. Obviously, the body's response to an absence of these estrogen foods produced symptoms identical to the withdrawal of synthetic estrogen. on the following page is a list of plant foods containing higher amounts of sterols, which are estrogen-like compounds. Including these foods regularly in the diet, following the principles of the 3-C Program and other suggestions listed will make coping with menopause much easier.

FOODS HIGH IN ESTROGEN-LIKE PLANT STEROLS

BEANS	WHOLE GRAINS	SEEDS	NUTS	OTHERS
Soybeans	**ALL** Except	Sesame	Coconut	Food Yeast
Calabar	rye, buckwheat	Sunflower	Peanuts	
	and white rice			

VEGETABLES	FRUITS	HERBS
Beets	Apples	Alfalfa
Brussel Sprouts	Cherries	Anise Seed
Carrots	Figs	Garlic
Corn (certain strains)	Lemon Peelings	Licorice Root
Eggplant	Olives	Oregano
Okra	Plums	Parsley
Peppers	Pomegranate	Red Raspberry
Potatoes	Strawberry	Sage
Radish Greens		
Seedlings:		
—Dry Barley		
—Common Bean		
—Pea		
Tomatoes		
Yams		

* For certain conditions, such as breast cancer, a diet low in plant sterols is advised. Check with a health professional.

—Exercise is as important as diet in dealing with menopause. In natural menopause, exercise is actually capable of stimulating the ovaries to produce *estrogen*. In the absence of ovaries, vigorous exercise can stimulate the adrenal glands to produce estrogen-like hormones. A proper exercise program (as described in Chapter 4) should gradually work up to one full hour. In some instances exercising for more than one hour may be necessary to alleviate symptoms.

—Fresh air and sunshine are especially important in controlling symptoms of menopause. The sun, which helps to promote Vitamin D production in the body, is actually a hormone that can also promote other hormone production.

—Water may also be used to stimulate the ovaries by use of a daily hot sitz bath for about one month. Hot compresses to the lower abdomen can also be helpful.

—Though it may sound minor, how a person dresses can affect the function of the body. It is helpful to avoid tight clothing and keep all parts of the body equally warm at all times. Chilling, especially of the hands, arms, feet and legs, can actually affect organs in the pelvic area.

If one has been faithfully following the recommendations of the 3-C Program for some time and is still having a particularly difficult time during menopause, there are several herbs (or herbal teas) that can provide safer alternatives to estrogen therapy. Consult a master herbalist, keep the treatment program simple by avoiding formulas containing multiple herbs, and build up slowly. Remember that herbs can be dangerous when used in conjunction with medicine.

Osteoporosis

More women die from fractures caused by osteoporosis than from cancer of the breast, cervix, and uterus combined. In the United States, hip-fracture health care costs up to $10 billion annually, and hip fractures lead to 200,000 deaths annually. That's 1 out of every 10 deaths.

What is osteoporosis, and what causes it? Osteoporosis is a condition of too-little bone mass or thinning of the bones. The chemical composition of the bone that exists is normal, but because there is less bone mass, the bones become brittle, weak, and more susceptible to fracture.

Bone is in a constant state of change, a process known as "remodeling." Small quantities of old bone are lost through resorption (broken down and absorbed) while at the same time new bone formation occurs. In osteoporosis, the formation of bone does not keep pace with its resorption. Some bone loss occurs universally with aging, especially in females. In an advanced state, bone loss can lead to primary osteoporosis. Secondary osteoporosis refers to bone loss associated with some other known cause, usually drug therapy or disease. In this case, bone loss is increased since it is superimposed on that of normal aging.

Inadequate bone density is most common in older women; however, it has also been found in women of 17 and 18 who consume average to high levels of dairy products. Even though the producers of dairy products insist that simply increasing calcium intake through dairy products will protect from, or at least retard osteoporosis, this is simply not the case. According to Dr. Gail Dalsky, PhD, the effectiveness of calcium alone in either maintaining or increasing bone mass has not been proven.

Research from other sources is rapidly uncovering some surprising facts about the true causes and prevention of osteoporosis. For example, attendees at the 1988 International Symposium on Osteoporosis found that many populations consume less calcium than Americans, yet show no signs of osteoporosis. They concluded that a low-calcium intake does not necessarily compromise bone composition. Other researchers state that although calcium is necessary for life itself, increasing calcium intake does nothing to contribute to laying down of bone, maintaining the skeleton, or to mending broken bones. Since there are potential hazards associated with calcium overload and taking calcium supplements, what can be done to avoid or slow down the progression of osteoporosis?

Diet plays an all-important role in making sure calcium requirements are met. Abundant calcium intake can be achieved through foods that do not pose the risk of dairy products (See food chart in this chapter, Calcium). Likewise, there are components other than calcium that aid in the prevention of bone loss. While calcium provides the hardness necessary for bone formation, other food components are essential in preventing bone loss. Collagen helps to provide tough connective tissue, while silicon chemically binds the structures of surface tissues and those that connect the bone. In primitive societies that have fewer incidence of osteoporosis, higher amounts of silicon are consumed. How can silicon be obtained? It can be found in unrefined, high-fiber foods such as brown rice, leafy greens, bell peppers, and others. Unfortunately, this vital component is lost in the typical processing of refined foods. Magnesium and boron are two other substances that seem to help in the fight against osteoporosis and are also available from a healthy diet of whole foods.

Information from various studies in recent years provides evidence that exercise is just as important as diet in the treatment and prevention of osteoporosis. In fact, one study by Dr. Dalsky showed that *exercise is more effective than calcium and estrogen supplements at increasing bone mass levels*. The benefits of exercise begin immediately; however, it may take some months to actually improve or increase bone density. One study showed that lumbar bone mineral content can increase significantly after only nine months of exercise. However, it is important that the type of exercise performed is a *weight-bearing exercise* (any exercise during which the body supports its own weight) such as jogging, walking, cycling, tennis, stair climbing, or aerobics. Walking combined with a minimal weight-lifting program seems to provide an excellent means of retaining bone mass.

Osteoporosis is a progressive, multifactorial, lifestyle-related disease. Concentrating on one factor to prevent the disease would be like focusing on a lower cholesterol level to avoid heart disease. Instead, eating a wholesome diet, exercising properly and consistently, and obtaining sunshine as much as possible (since Vitamin D helps to utilize calcium) will go a long way toward the prevention and treatment of this disease.

Allergies

An allergy is an altered capacity to react. The substance to which a person reacts differently is called an allergen, or antigen. There are hundreds of allergens, but many Candida patients commonly have allergies to foods, dusts, pollens, molds, and mildew.

Aside from these common allergies, some Candida patients have "uncommon" allergies to medications, chemicals, or synthetics in the environment. They, like the author once was, are often considered "chemically or environmentally" sensitive to modern-day chemicals and experience allergic reactions ranging from mild to life-threatening. The 3-C Program has been very successful in helping alleviate allergies of all types. Experience has shown that the average recovery time for food allergies is normally 60 to 90 days. Chemical or environmental allergies may take a little longer. Below are a few suggestions and some review from previous chapters pertinent to dealing with allergies.

—The body reacts in an allergic manner when it cannot tolerate a particular substance. Therefore, in the beginning of the 3-C Program, it may be necessary to avoid contact with known allergens. This is easily accomplished with food since one can simply leave certain foods out of the diet for the first few weeks of the program. Then, try those foods again every few weeks and watch closely for a reaction.

—Staying clear of environmental or chemical allergens is more difficult than avoiding food. In this instance, a person can only control her (or his) environment as best she (or he) can and continue the program faithfully. The overwhelming majority of environmentally-sensitive Candida patients are able to recover in their own homes by simply following the program. Very rarely does a person have to change environments (such as relocating for a short time) to limit exposure to reactive substances that constantly challenge the immune system. In this instance, a short time away from the source of allergens can allow the immune system the chance it needs to rebuild itself.

—It is extremely helpful to keep a journal, recording diet and amounts of 3-C Helpers taken. This is only necessary in the beginning of the program when allergies are still a problem. Since it is frustrating trying to figure out whether one is experiencing an allergic reaction or die-off, journal entries help pinpoint the cause. For instance, if a garlic dosage was just increased, adverse symptoms could be due to die-off rather than an allergy. On the other hand, if a new food was introduced that same day, the symptoms could stem from an actual intolerance to that food.

—A properly functioning digestive system is imperative to a strong immune system. So that digestion of all food is efficient, carefully observe every single digestion principle listed in Chapter 3, so that digestion of all food is efficient.

—Remember that a strong immune system better tolerates allergens. Even though all components of this program will help to rebuild the immune system, exercise is especially beneficial in accomplishing this. In fact, there have been several incidents in which Candida patients were following the program faithfully and were very happy to find their allergies disappearing. Assuming it would not hurt to discontinue only the exercise portion of the program for a few days, they were alarmed to discover allergic symptoms returning. As soon as they added exercise back into their program, they began feeling better. The moral of the story is: Exercise plays a crucial role in Candida recovery.

In summary, allergies indicate that there is a weakness in the immune system that needs to be strengthened. The 3-C Program, faithfully followed, can help to restore both systems.

Medications

Wouldn't it be nice if all health problems could be remedied by taking a pill? Especially if that pill, after working its "magic," would exit the body leaving no trace of damage behind? Unfortunately, this is not the way it works. Every chemical taken into the body has an affect on the body. The results of harmful chemicals can remain in the body for a long time, as any pathologist can verify. Naturally, the extent of damage will depend on many factors, including what chemical or medication was used, how much and for how long, as well as individual tolerances. Therefore, the 3-C Program does not recommend the use of chemical medications.

Even though drug medications do have a place in emergencies or exceptional situations, most often nature has provided alternatives that can facilitate in healing, eliminating long-term damage to the body. For instance, the drug nystatin, typically used in Candida treatment programs, is an anti-fungal medication that has been shown to reduce yeast. However, it is a mold-based, antibiotic medication. Although nystatin is not supposed to cause long-range damage to the body, it has been shown to cause side effects in some people. It is also expensive and often is only effective for a period of time, as is common with many antibiotic medications to which the body eventually develops an immunity. Alternately, the *Kyolic* liquid garlic product recommended in the 3-C Program is a natural product that encourages one's own immune system to reduce yeast colonization, resulting in better overall health. It also costs less than nystatin. Many real-life experiences have shown that one's immune system can recover much more quickly and thoroughly without the use of drug medications. Therefore, if you are taking a medication that is not absolutely necessary, consider discontinuing it after checking with one's health professional. If you are taking a life-saving medication, continue on it and advise the health professional about one's lifestyle changes. Certainly, most health professionals who would take the time to study this program, though perhaps not agreeing with all the principles, would acknowledge that it is an all-natural health recovery program that does not advocate harmful or extreme doctrine.

Cravings

Candida patients typically complain of cravings, especially for foods containing yeast or sugar. For many, cravings are a struggle of the mind as well as the body. Often, they are told that their desire to eat is due to a lack of will power and can be controlled. While there is the possibility that being preoccupied with food and overeating has become a habit that must be broken, it is not true that cravings are a sign of weak willpower. Cravings are a real, physical symptom of Candida created by yeast organisms.

Cravings can also be accentuated by a diet low in wholesome foods that does not support blood sugar levels between meals. Diets consisting of refined, processed, nutrient-deficient food allow the blood sugar to drop, causing feelings of hunger, as well as other hypoglycemic symptoms. Foods such as sugar, milk, cheese, eggs, meats, salt and chemicals such as caffeine and nicotine are known to promote cravings.

Many health professionals advise eating often during the day and evening to "keep up the blood sugar." However, as shown in Chapter 3, it is obvious that eating between meals is a lifestyle choice that **delays** digestion, causing fermentation, which encourages yeast. Fermentation and eating fermented foods causes irritation of the nerves of the stomach. These nerves then send out *signals of hunger*. Therefore, eating only at specified mealtimes and avoiding fermented, spicy, and salty foods will help eliminate cravings.

Once again, it may take a good dose of will power to cope with cravings in the beginning of the program. Until the regulating benefits of the program have reduced cravings, try the suggestions below at the first sign of cravings:

—Drinking a glass of cold water can displace cravings. Since dehydration encourages cravings, it is vital to consume adequate water every day.

—Because exercise helps to curb hunger, taking a brisk walk outside in the fresh air is an excellent aid. During working hours or whenever time is limited, even a few minutes spent deeply breathing fresh air can rejuvenate and take one's mind off food. Diversion tactics are also helpful, such as going to visit a friend, working in the garden, or shopping.

—If it is not possible to go outside, try to do something inside that is not associated with food, such as a hobby or cleaning. Calling a friend or family member for support is ideal *only if* that person is understanding and supportive. (Too often, the validity of this illness is challenged by those who should be the greatest supporters. In this case, avoid those people or do not bring up the subject of one's illness.)

The battle with cravings is not normally a long one. Most symptoms subside in a few weeks, providing many Candida patients with control over this situation for the first time in years.

Overweight

A great many Candida patients are unhappy with their weight. Typically, more of them are overweight than underweight. Below are suggestions to deal with both problems.

The 3-C Diet is largely comprised of complex carbohydrate foods which are readily assimilated and utilized. For this reason, overweight people most always notice a weight loss that begins within a few weeks. Likewise, the *Kyolic* liquid garlic seems to encourage regulation of the thyroid, aiding in weight-balancing. Even overweight people not participating in the 3-C Program find the *Kyolic* liquid garlic beneficial in weight loss. The combination of the 3-C Diet, exercise, water, and garlic will reduce fat, increase lean muscle, and help one feel wonderful. However, two of these factors work in a way that are surprising.

First of all, *exercising early in the morning* increases the body's metabolism, causing the body to burn calories at nearly twice the rate for the next six to eight hours. Think about that. Exercise gears up the body's metabolism and increases its ability to "burn" calories. Exercise should be a main component in any weight-loss program.

Second, the 3-C principle of "eating breakfast like a king, lunch like a prince, and supper like a pauper" will accomplish more than just ensuring a person is well-fed. Many people feel that eating a large breakfast will only add unnecessary calories, causing weight gain. What they do not realize is that *skipping breakfast will slow down weight loss* by lowering metabolism and robbing the body of needed nutrients.

Similarly, going light on lunch, especially after skipping breakfast, is like putting the body through a daily fast, which again lowers metabolism and intensifies the effects of poor nutrition. It is easy to see that a lowered metabolism and poor nutrition accelerate hypoglycemic conditions, causing a lack of necessary energy and nutrients to complete afternoon and early evening activity. The result is a person who may feel irritable and overwhelmed by even simple demands of the afternoon and evening (i.e. coping with work in the afternoon, fixing dinner, or dealing with children). No wonder people feel overwhelmed. The brain is being denied the glucose it needs to think, reason, and coordinate the body's responses to normal activity. Eating whole foods, on a regular basis, will actually aid in weight loss.

If, in the beginning of the 3-C Program one is inclined to overeat, below are some tips to help resist the urge. (Before long, control of the appetite is regained and one finds satisfaction in eating a normal, healthy amount of food).

—Even though raw foods will be avoided the first few weeks on this program, they will soon be added to the diet. Raw foods should always be the first eaten at a meal, prior to cooked foods. Besides being filling, the natural digestive enzymes in raw foods are beneficial to digestion.

—Enough food should be eaten to *satisfy hunger, not appetite.* One should feel comfortably full, but not stuffed.

—A glass of water one-half hour before a meal helps curb appetite, but remember that fluids directly before or with a meal will dilute digestive enzymes and inhibit proper digestion. Making sure that the daily water requirement is met is also important in appetite control.

—Meals should be relaxing and unhurried. Take small bites, chew slowly and *thoroughly.* It takes 20 minutes for the satiety center in the brain to register the effects of the first stage of digestion. If food is "gulped," a larger amount of it will be eaten before the feeling of satisfaction is registered. Also, "chunks" of food are more difficult to digest.

—Putting only as much food as should be eaten on one's plate, with no refills, is a good rule of thumb. It may even be necessary to leave the kitchen immediately after eating to stay away from food. Many people find that brushing their teeth helps them forget about the taste of the food.

Although less common than being overweight, being underweight is just as frustrating for some Candida patients. In an attempt to gain weight, many Candida patients are overeating meat products, having been told they will provide protein for weight gain yet not encourage yeast growth. Realistically, meat provides an overabundance of protein that is low in fiber and nutrients and does nothing to correct the problem of malabsorption so common in underweight people. When beginning the 3-C Program, it is not unusual to lose a few pounds, especially when eliminating meat from the diet. However, there is no cause for alarm as long as all foods from the Getting Well diet are used. After losing a few pounds, most people find that their weight stabilizes for a time, and then they begin to gain weight. Remember, it is much better to be thin and healthy than to be heavy and unhealthy. If all principles of the 3-C Program are carefully followed, a person will not only feel good, but will eventually look healthy. It will simply take some time. These suggestions may help:

—Surprisingly, exercising everyday is beneficial. Even though exercise may speed up metabolism, it also promotes good digestion. If one is not absorbing nutrients from food, it is very difficult to gain weight.

—Water is instrumental in transporting nutrients from food to each cell of the body. So, be certain to drink the required amount of water every single day.

—Chew food slowly and well! Chewing food is the first stage of digestion. If it is not completed properly, neither will any other stage of digestion.

—Giving up meat does not mean giving up calories. Simply consuming extra amounts of beans and whole grains usually helps. For example, if you are eating approximately one cup of beans at a meal, increase that portion by a half-cup or more. Do the same with the whole grains. Continue with these amounts over the next couple of months. Experience has shown that specifically including garbanzo beans, millet, avocados, and seeds in the diet several times a week is especially helpful in gaining weight. However, since avocados and seeds are concentrated, make certain not to over-do on them. Once again, eating too much food will not accomplish weight gain since an overloaded digestive system cannot efficiently break down and absorb nutrients.

—Regularity is crucial in gaining weight, as well as in good health. All principles of the 3-C Program need to be utilized on a regular basis, strictly following the daily schedule. Plenty of sleep at regular times is especially important when attempting to gain weight.

Gas/Indigestion

Many Candida patients have intestinal problems, such as flatulence (gas), indigestion, or bloating. When intestinal gas is formed, acids are often produced, which causes colon discomfort. In the beginning of this program, die-off may increase intestinal gas. However, as digestion improves, intestinal difficulties should subside. Simply becoming a vegetarian will help, since fats and proteins derived from eating meat and other animal by-products are the major carriers of odor residues. Carbohydrates provided by the 3-C Diet are mostly the odorless components of intestinal gas, with the exception of beans. However, if beans are properly cooked and if the digestive system has had some time to improve, intestinal gas should be a problem of the past. The suggestions below may help.

Every bite of food should be chewed to a "cream" consistency before swallowing since the first stage of digestion occurs in the mouth.

Mealtimes should last approximately 30 to 40 minutes. Eating too fast or too slow can encourage intestinal gas.

Enough food should be consumed to be comfortably full, not stuffed.

There should be at least five hours from the end of one meal until the beginning of the next.

Meals should be eaten at regular times every day.

Fruits and vegetables should not be eaten at the same meal.

Known allergic foods should be left out of the diet until the digestive system has improved.

No liquids, in any form, should be consumed with meals. Fruit juices and other foods high in water volume can also create gas.

Plenty of water is needed between meals.

Stress during mealtimes can delay digestion and produce gas.

Dried beans and whole grains should be thoroughly cooked.

Reclining after meals slows digestion. Light activity is ideal.

Miscellaneous Illness

Most people implementing health recovery programs that utilize the 3-C principles do so in an effort to rectify their Candida problem. However, it has often been the case that many other conditions were improved by these same principles. Among these were various illnesses such as Epstein-Barr (sometimes referred to as Chronic Fatigue Syndrome), lupus, arthritis, cancer, multiple sclerosis, and muscular dystrophy. Improvements in other conditions, such as thyroid problems, tachycardia, diabetes, kidney disease, hypertension and cardiovascular disease, have also been apparent.

The credit for improvement in certain conditions lies in the principles of a good health recovery program. Becoming a strict vegetarian does not mean one will become nutrient-deficient in the process. A quote from the American Dietetic Association says, "The Dietary Guidelines for Americans recommends a reduction in fat intake and an increased consumption of fruits, vegetables and whole grains. Well-planned vegetarian diets effectively meet these guidelines and the Recommended Dietary Allowances can be confidently embraced as a healthy dietary alternative. Vegetarians are at lower risk for noninsulin-dependent diabetes and have lower rates of hypertension, osteoporosis, kidney stones, gallstones and diverticular disease than nonvegetarians." Studies show that vegetarians consuming a healthy variety of plant foods typically do not suffer the tremendous amount of degenerative diseases that plague nonvegetarians.

SUMMARY OF DIGESTION PRINCIPLES

Chew Food Well
Eat Two Or Three Meals A Day With Nothing Between
Liquids Should Not Be Consumed With Meals
Eliminate Eating In The Evenings
Reduce Number Of Foods At Each Meal
Practice Simple Food Combining
Limit Refined And Concentrated Foods
Utilize Proper Exercise At Proper Times
Control Stres

CHAPTER 9

GETTING WELL RECIPES

Many of the recipes listed in this section are comprised of very few ingredients, as recommended in Getting Well. However, to provide a little variety, there are some that contain slightly more than three or four ingredients. One should wait to try these recipes until they have made some progress. Until then, simply eat from the simple food groups described in Chapter 6, using the recipes that have fewer ingredients.

As improvement comes, one can try the recipes that contain one or more extra ingredients, watching carefully for any adverse reactions.

BEANS (LEGUMES)

Many people feel they cannot tolerate the indigestion and intestinal gas normally associated with eating beans. However, the cooking method described below will aid in breaking down gas-forming starches and render beans' nutrients easier to assimilate. Though this process may seem slightly lengthy at first, the results are worth the effort. Eventually, beans may be tolerated after only two short-boils; however, this should only be tried after recovery. Do not be concerned that long cooking times will reduce the nutrient value of beans. The chart shows that the loss of nutrients is very minimal.

NUTRIENT RETENTION OF BEANS (LEGUMES)
(After 2 1/2 Hours of Cooking)

NUTRIENT	PERCENT RETENTION
Calcium	90
Iron	80
Magnesium	75
Phosphorus	85
Potassium	70
Sodium	95
Zinc	90
Copper	60
Manganese	80
Ascorbic acid	70
Thiamin	45
Riboflavin	80
Niacin	60
Pantothenic acid	55
Vitamin B$_6$	55
Folacin	35
Vitamin A	90

COOKING BEANS

Step 1 - Soaking

Rinse and sort the beans, picking out any discolored or shriveled ones. Put in a large pot with three or four times their volume of water and cover. (In warm weather, soak beans in refrigerator to prevent fermenting.) Soaking beans for at least eight hours is a very important aspect of the preparation process: not only are the beans easier to cook to a soft consistency, but in the soaking process the dormant life force of the bean is activated. If beans are needed in a hurry, bring them with water to a boil. Then turn off heat and let them set, covered, for one hour. Continue with other steps. Beans such as lentils, mung, and split peas do not require soaking. Start the cooking process for them with Step 2. One cup of dry beans will yield approximately 2 1/2 cups of cooked beans.

Step 2 - Short Boils

Put soaked, drained beans into fresh, clean water. Bring to a boil on stovetop and continue to boil for approximately 10 minutes. Repeat this process two more times, changing water each time. *you will boil the beans for 10 minutes each time in clean, fresh water for a total of three times.* Boil the beans for 10 minutes each time in clean, fresh water for a total of three times. During each subsequent boiling, less dark foam should appear. Now, the beans should have released most of the gaseous starches.

Step 3 - Long Boil

In clean, fresh water, bring the beans to a low boil on the stovetop until they are completely cooked, usually several hours for most beans. *Make certain the beans are completely and thoroughly cooked.* Beans should mash very easily between fingers when done. (See chart below.)

Tips For Cooking Beans

—Seasonings such as garlic, onions, or mild herbs can be added at the beginning of the cooking stage or shortly before the beans finish cooking. Salt, however, should be added near the end of cooking time since it tends to toughen the skins and lengthens cooking time.

—Avoid consuming too much liquid with prepared beans. Simply pour off excess liquid, freeze, and use it for soup stock (or can be fed to pets).

—Pureed beans are very versatile. They can be added to any recipe to thicken or bind.

3-C BEAN (LEGUMES) COOKING CHART

BEAN (1 cup dry)	WATER	COOKING TIME (LONG-BOILS)	YIELD
Black Beans	4 cups	90 minutes	2 cups
Black-eyed Peas	3 cups	60 minutes	2 cups
Garbanzos (Chick Peas)	4 cups	3 hours	2 cups
Great Northern	4 cups	2 hours	2 cups
Kidney Beans	3 cups	90 minutes	2 cups
Lentils & Split Peas	3 cups	60 minutes	2 cups
Limas	2 cups	90 minutes	1 cup
Baby Limas	2 cups	90 minutes	2 cups
Pinto Beans	3 cups	3 hours	2 cups
Red Beans	3 cups	3 hours	2 cups
Sm. White Beans (navy, etc.)	3 cups	2 hours	2 cups
Soybeans	4 cups	3 hours	2 cups
Soy Grits	2 cups	15 minutes	2 cups

CrockPot Cooking

Most people find the easiest method of cooking beans is to substitute crock-pot cooking for stovetop cooking. However, the crock-pot method, while more convenient, does take longer since most crock-pots do not reach a high temperature. Most instructions call for using three or four parts water to one part beans. Since we are attempting to consume the least amount of water possible with our food, use three parts water to one part beans. Using this method, most beans should cook approximately 12 hours (on high). This method works especially well if beans are soaked overnight, short-boiled three times in the morning and then left cooking all day.

Oven Cooking

A variation of crockpot cooking is oven cooking. After three short-boils, simply use three parts water to one part beans. Bring to boil on stovetop using oven-proof pot. Cover and place in 200 degree oven for approximately 8-10 hours.

Pressure Cooking

Pressure cooking reduces cooking time and is not dangerous if the manufacturer's instructions are closely followed. The main consideration with cooking beans in a pressure cooker is making sure the vents do not clog with foam. Certain beans (split peas, lima beans, fava beans, and soybeans) are not recommended for pressure cooking because of excessive foaming. Most other beans should do fine. Just remember to follow Steps 1 and 2 and to cook them thoroughly (which will be longer than the recommended manufacturer's cooking time). Do not remove lid until pressure gauge has been released, all steam has escaped, and the valve or steam indicator shows all pressure is reduced.

SPROUTING

Very rarely will a person experience gas after the 3-C cooking process. If so, one would benefit from eating sprouted beans at first. Follow Step 1 – Soaking. Drain and rinse beans and follow your preferred sprouting method. A simple one to use is: Take a half-gallon jar and lay on its side. Spread a cup of rinsed beans inside, place a piece of cheesecloth over opening and put a jar ring over. Cover with a towel to keep dark. Rinse and drain twice a day in cool/normal weather and three times a day in hot weather. Re-spread and cover again. After two days, remove towel and place jar in sun to develop the chlorophyll. The sprouts growing out of the beans should be approximately 1/4 to 1/2 inch long. Rinse well, discarding any unsprouted beans. The sprouting process will increase the vitamin content, as well as making the beans more digestible.

BEAN RECIPES

BAKED BEANS
6 C any cooked bean
1/2 C tomato sauce or 1 C tomatoes
1 C water
1 T lemon juice
1 onion, chopped
1 sm. clove garlic, chopped
Salt to taste

Mix and place in a bean pot or baking dish. Bake at 350 degrees for 1 hour or longer.

BLACK-EYED PEA LOAF

2 C black-eyed peas, cooked
2 C water
1 lg. onion, chopped
2 t favorite herbs
1/3 C rolled oats
1 1/2 C corn meal
Salt to taste

Blend first five ingredients in blender. Pour into corn meal and mix. Bake in a loaf pan at 350 degrees for 1 1/2 hours. The darker brown it gets, the more firm the slices become, to the point that the slices may be used as corn bread.

ENCHILADAS

3 C cooked beans with one cup liquid from beans
1 C cooked brown rice
1 t onion powder
1 t garlic powder
1 t salt
1 t paprika
Tomato sauce
Tortillas

Mix thoroughly all ingredients, heat and put in middle of the tortilla. Wrap tortilla and place (seam side down) in a baking dish spread with tomato sauce on the bottom. Cover with more tomato sauce. Bake 40-50 minutes at 325 degrees or until hot.

CHICKEN-STYLE RICE

2 C cooked garbanzo (chickpea) beans
2 C brown rice, raw
2 C canned tomatoes
4 onions, sliced
4 C water
2 t salt
1 t basil

Mix all ingredients in a three quart casserole. Cover and bake at 325 degrees for 2-3 hours, adding more tomato juice if necessary. May be cooked on top of stove if desired, but do not stir after the first 20 minutes as the rice gets sticky.

CREOLE
1/2 C hot water
1 1/4 C diced onion
2 tomatoes, fresh or canned, peeled and diced
1 bay leaf
2 t salt
1/2 C tomato sauce
3 C cooked garbanzos
Hot brown rice, cooked

Sauté onion in water in a large skillet over low heat until tender. Add tomatoes, bay leaf, salt, and tomato sauce. Cover and simmer 15 minutes. Add garbanzos. Cover and simmer 10 minutes longer. Serve over brown rice.

MEXICAN BEAN SOUP
2 C pinto or garbanzo (chickpea) beans
2 onions, diced
2 cloves garlic, diced
1/2 C tomato sauce
Salt as needed

Cook beans with onions and garlic according to 3-C Chart. Fifteen minutes before end of cooking time, mix in the tomato sauce and salt.

CONNIE'S RED LENTIL SOUP
1 C dry red lentils
2 pkgs frozen chopped spinach or equivalent fresh
2 T chopped onion
1 1/2 t dried parsley
1/2 t dried basil
Salt to taste

Cook lentils according to 3-C Chart, adding spinach, onion, parsley, and basil. Add salt to taste shortly before finished cooking time.

BAKED LENTILS
3 C lentils
1/4 C onions, diced
2 C tomatoes
2 t salt
1/2 C bread crumbs (recipe in Grain section)

Cook lentils and onions according to 3-C Chart, adding salt near end of cooking time. Blend tomatoes in blender and heat just to boiling. Add to lentils. There should be no excess water in lentils. Place all in a baking dish, topping with bread crumbs. Bake until crumbs are a golden brown.

LENTIL PATTIES

2 C lentils, cooked
3 C finely ground bread crumbs (recipe in Grain section)
1 onion, diced
1 t salt
1 C water (or more)
2 T parsley, chopped

Mix all ingredients and form into patties. Place on floured cookie sheet. Bake at 350 degrees for 20 to 30 minutes or until nicely browned. Makes 10-15 patties.

LENTIL POT

2 C lentils
1 C tomatoes
1 C chopped onions
1 bay leaf
1 T lemon juice, optional
Salt as needed

Cook lentils according to 3-C chart. Adding remaining ingredients approximately 1/2 hour before end of cooking time. Excellent over rice or potatoes. Makes about 3 1/2 cups.

TOSTADO FILLING

2 onions, chopped
1 t garlic powder
2 C tomatoes, chopped
2 t salt
8 C cooked beans
Tostados

Sauté onions in water, add next 3 ingredients and cook for 15 minutes. Add beans and simmer another 15 minutes. Can be blended again for a smoother consistency. Serve over tostadoes or any bread or cracker item; top with chopped lettuce and tomatoes. Can be kept hot in oven for serving.

BEANS (LEGUMES)

VICKI'S BEAN BURRITOS

4 C cooked beans (such as pintos)
2 1/2 C tomatoes, chopped
1 C bell pepper, chopped
1 C onion, chopped
2 t celery salt
Burritos

Mix all ingredients and simmer slowly about 45 minutes. Fill burritos and serve with rice, or mix rice into mixture and fill burritos. Also can be used as a side dish.

WHOLE GRAINS

Purchasing And Storing Whole Grains

Whole grains can be purchased at most health food stores. However, better pricing can normally be found at bulk food or health food co-op stores. If a co-op store is not available, one can advertise to join a co-op group where people combine orders to take advantage of bulk food buying. Usually, these orders will be delivered to one person, who breaks the larger quantities into smaller ones, then contacts the members to pick up their merchandise. Even though more expensive, there are several reputable companies who offer whole grain products through catalogues. Whatever the source, try to purchase the freshest grain possible.

Grain is best stored in the freezer or in bug-proof containers in a cool, dry area. One method that the author used was a "dry canning" method, which was passed on from the Amish community. Although this method is not typically used today (the County Extension agents could not locate its use in their records), the author has successfully preserved grain in this method for up to four years.

Dry Canning Method: Place the *dry* grain in a clean, *dry* glass canning jar. Apply a new lid since this method will actually produce a seal. Place the ring around the lid. After filling all desired jars, place them standing up in a preheated 250-degree oven. The entire rack may be filled, leaving only a slight space between jars. Close the oven door and *do not open it*. After 45 minutes, simply turn the oven off. *Again, do not open the door, for the sealing occurs from the progressive, uninterrupted cooling of the oven.* Leave the jars in the oven overnight (or for a minimum of eight hours). Then, remove jars from oven; they should be sealed. Store jars in a cool, dark place. Remember, if the grain is washed before canning, spread it out and dry it thoroughly before canning. (The grain can also be washed after canning and prior to cooking.)

Flours and cracked grain products need to be refrigerated or frozen immediately after milling. Flour can be refrigerated for short periods, such as a week or two, or frozen for up to several months in order to prevent oxidation/rancidity, which starts immediately after milling.

Cooking Whole Grains

Whole grain kernels, or "berries," in most instances refers to grain in its natural state as it comes out of the field, with only the outermost, hard covering removed. Before cooking whole grain berries, first spread them out on a large surface and sort through, removing any stones, dirt or foreign objects. Rinse under running water in a strainer, turning grain over several times. If grain is then going to be cooked into a cereal, proceed with cooking methods listed below. If grain is to be ground into flour, it is important not to put it into the mill (grinding device) damp because the moisture could possibly damage the mill. Instead, spread the grain out on a countertop, cookie sheet, wax paper, or towels, until dry. Then it can be ground into flour.

Keep in mind that although some foods, such as most vegetables, are more nourishing if they have a shorter cooking time, other foods, such as beans, whole grains, and starchy vegetables have nutrients that are difficult to obtain *unless they are thoroughly cooked*. Thorough cooking helps to split or break down the molecules in these foods, a task that is very difficult for the digestive system to accomplish. Undercooked beans, whole grains, and starchy vegetables can result in indigestion, gas, or an overall intolerance to these foods. Therefore, the recommended cooking times in the 3-C Program will definitely be longer than any other recommendations one may have previously encountered.

Other methods that can aid in grain tolerability are: 1) to cook whole grains for 10 minutes, then throw off the water. Put whole grains in a pot of clean, fresh water and continue with the desired cooking method; 2) to dextrinize grain as described below, and 3) to sprout grain, also described below.

It is not necessary to be concerned about nutrient loss when cooking whole grains for long periods of time since the majority of nutrients are lost only in the first ten minutes of cooking.

Dextrinizing Whole Grains

While it is not absolutely necessary to dextrinize whole grains, it is very helpful. Dextrinizing is a process used prior to cooking that gives whole grains a sweeter flavor as well as rendering it more easily digested.

Technically speaking, dextrinizing changes the long-chain car-bohydrates in grain to short-chain carbohydrates. To dextrinize (some-times referred to as "browning") whole or "cracked" grain berries, simply heat either wet or dry grain in a dry skillet, stirring constantly on moderate heat for three to five minutes. Be careful not to burn! Dextrinizing can also be accomplished in the oven by baking the grain berries in a dry pan for five to ten minutes at 325 degrees. Whole-grain flour can also be dextrinized on the stovetop or in the oven, similar to whole grain berries, except that the heat should be lowered and extra caution be used so the flour does not burn!

As discussed in length in Chapter 5, it is most beneficial to consume whole grains in one of three ways: cooked into a cereal, freshly ground into a flour and then cooked, or sprouted. Cooking methods for each of these is discussed below.

Methods For Cooking Whole Grains Into Cereal:

1. Stovetop Method: Bring salted water (see cooking chart that follows) to a boil. Add the grain while stirring. Return to a boil, lower the heat, and simmer, covered, for the recommended time.

3-C COOKING CHART FOR WHOLE GRAINS

GRAIN (1 CUP DRY)	WATER	COOKING TIME
Barley, hulled	3 Cups	1-2 Hours
Buckwheat Groats	2-3 Cups	1-2 Hours
Cornmeal	4 Cups	45-60 Minutes
Millet, hulled	3-4 Cups	90 Minutes
Oats, Whole (Oat Groats)	3-4 Cups	2-3 Hours
Steel-Cut Oats	3-4 Cups	90 Minutes
Rolled (Oatmeal)	2-3 Cups	60 Minutes
Rice, Brown (Fluffy)		
short	2 1/2 Cups	60 Minutes
medium	2 Cups	60 Minutes
long	1 1/2 Cups	60 Minutes

For creamier rice, add more water

Rye Berries	3 Cups	2 Hours
Wheat Berries	3 Cups	2 Hours
Cracked Wheat	2-3 Cups	60 Minutes

If "fluffier" whole grains are desired, it is best not to lift the lid or stir them. However, if a a "creamy" texture is desired, stir whole grains a couple of times during the cooking process.

Leftover whole grains can easily be reheated without drying by simply steaming in a steamer or double boiler for a short time.

WHOLE GRAINS

2. Overnight Stovetop Method: Bring salted water to a boil. Add whole grains and simmer, covered, for one hour. Remove from heat and let stand overnight. In the morning, bring grain to a boil again and cook on low boil for 30 to 60 minutes or until tender. Or, place in oven at 350 degrees for one hour. This method works especially well for wheat, rye, and oat berries.

3. Oven Method: Place grain, water, and salt into a casserole dish. Stir briefly to mix in the salt. Bake at 200 degrees overnight. Grain will be ready to serve in the morning. It can also be baked at a higher temperature (350 degrees) for several hours rather than overnight.

4. Crockpot Method: Place grain, water, and salt in crockpot. Stir briefly to mix salt. Cook on high for several hours and then on low overnight. Cereal will be ready to eat in the morning. If one experiences problems when eating grain prepared in the crockpot, try another method of cooking.

5. Pressure Cooking Method: This method requires less water and is faster than regular cooking, requiring less energy and preparation. Because each brand of pressure cooker varies, refer to the manufacturer's instructions carefully for proper use. A stainless steel pressure cooker is highly recommended over an aluminum one.

Cooking With Whole Grain Flour

It is important to remember that once a grain has been cracked or ground, oxidation begins immediately. After a few days at room temperature, grain flour will lose a good deal of its nutrients. That is why it is advisable to grind whole grains fresh. Flour from even a health food store is likely to be nutrient-deficient.

Whole-grain flour can be prepared into many different products, such as waffles, biscuits, grain cakes, chapatis, and muffins. (Refer to the recipe section.) Although whole-grain flour products do not need to be cooked as long as whole grains, it is still important to cook them well.

Bread and Cracker Crumbs

Recipes calling for bread or cracker crumbs can easily be made from virtually any dried grain item. For instance, hush puppies, corn fritters, chapatis, or easy oat crackers can be thoroughly dried in the oven and put into the blender to grind into fine crumbs. Or, leftover cooked grain can be spread on a cookie sheet, thoroughly dried in the oven, then ground in a blender.

Sprouting Whole Grains

Sprouting actually changes the molecular structure of grain, making it even easier to digest than other preparation methods do. Even though the other cooking methods normally conquer intolerance to grain, sprouting is ideal for very sensitive people. Or, sprouted whole grains can be added to any diet for a powerhouse of nutrition. Sprouting whole grains can be accomplished by:

Step 1. Soaking – Wash whole grains, throwing out any broken or undesirable pieces. Measure approximately two tablespoons of grain berries into a quart glass jar. Add a cup or so of warm water. Cover the jar opening with cheesecloth, clean nylon stocking, or fine-mesh screen. Hold in place with a rubber band or ring. Let soak for 8 to 12 hours. Drain off soaking water, rinsing berries with lukewarm water. Keep rinsing until the water runs clear. (The original soaking water is excellent for house plants.) Drain thoroughly.

Step 2. Rinsing and Draining – Place jar on its side with cheesecloth, stocking or screen over the mouth. Put in a warm (70 degrees) area away from direct sunlight. Rinse and drain the berries two or three times a day, more often in hot or humid weather. (The reason for the rinsing and draining is to promote sprouting without fermentation.) When the berries begin to sprout little "stems" about one-quarter of an inch long move the jar to a sunny area such as a sliding glass door or window sill. The light will make the sprout leaves turn green since light promotes beneficial chlorophyll.

Sprouts should be immediately refrigerated and used within one week. They will stay fresher a day or two longer if kept in a glass container rather than plastic. For those who love sprouting but are not home to rinse and drain, there are electric sprouters that require nothing

WHOLE GRAINS

more than to be filled with water and seeds, and then turned on. After approximately two days, a fresh crop of sprouts should be ready. (See Resource section.)

GRAIN RECIPES

BREAD REPLACEMENT IDEAS

SPROUTED GRAIN BREAD
1 C sprouted wheat berries
1 t salt
chopped seeds (optional)

Sprout 1 cup hard winter wheat berries for three days (1/4-1/2" long). Put 1 cup of sprouts into a blender and blend until creamy. Place in mixing bowl. Add 4 cups whole wheat flour (2 cups whole wheat and 2 cups whole wheat pastry flour works best), and 1 teaspoon salt, if desired. Chopped seeds are optional. Mix together and knead with floured hands. Put in a loaf pan or shape into a loaf on hard surface and cover with a damp cloth. Let rise naturally for 8-10 hours. Bake at 350 degrees for 1 hour. This is a substantial bread that remains chewy.

RICE BISCUITS
2 C cooked brown rice
1 scant t salt
1 1/3 C fine brown rice flour
1/2 C unhulled sesame seeds (optional)

Mash hot cooked brown rice with a fork, adding salt. Add brown rice flour and knead into a pliable dough. Roll out into a 1/2" thick square and cut into 2" squares. Place on a cookie sheet and bake at 375 degrees for 15 minutes. If necessary, turn over and bake 10 minutes longer or until golden brown. Rice biscuits should be soft inside but not doughy. These are best fresh. If frozen, reheat before serving by steaming until warm. Makes 24 biscuits.

VICKI'S GRAIN CAKES

These grain cakes can be made from any grain. A good one to start with is millet. Cook a batch of whole millet cereal according to 3-C directions. Place some type of a round mold, such as a Tupperware hamburger mold, or the rim that normally fits around a canning jar lid, on a non-stick cookie sheet (or dust cookie sheet with grain flour). Spoon the hot cooked millet into the mold and smooth flat on top. If the cooked grain sticks to the mold, dip mold in a pan of ice water between moldings.

Bake for 1 to 2 hours, at 200 degrees, until the cakes have "dried" to suit individual preference. A crunchy rice-cake result will require longer baking than a more moist cake. For example, if the cakes are still a little "doughy" in the middle, bake at a lower temperature for a longer period of time to remove the moisture from the cakes. These can be frozen and easily thawed by simply placing in a toaster. It may be necessary to experiment with baking times, depending on what type of cooked grain is used.

Certain whole grains that have a gelatinous quality, such as millet, oats, and barley, can be cooked and then put into the refrigerator in a mold (loaf pan, tube pan, etc.) until cold. Remove from mold, slice in 1/3 to 1/2" slices and bake in 350 degree oven for 45 to 60 minutes.

CHAPATIS
2 C whole grain flour
2 T seeds, ground
1 C water
1/2 t salt

Mix salt and water, then add to flour (add seeds if desired) and mix thoroughly. Dough should be stiff like a pastry dough. Add more flour if needed. Let dough sit for one-half hour. Divide dough into balls about the size of a small egg. Roll each ball out to about 6" in diameter. Bake chapatis about 1 1/2 hours in 250 degree oven, or over burner in heavy skillet, until brown.

EASY OAT CRACKERS
1 1/4 C quick or rolled oats
1/3 C whole wheat flour or any other whole grain flour
1 T wheat germ or raw bran
1/4 t salt
1/3 C cold water

Blend oats in blender until they are very fine. Pour into a mixing bowl, adding flour, wheat germ, and salt. Mix. Add water. Mix well

WHOLE GRAINS

again. Roll out onto a cookie sheet 1/8" thick. Score with the tines of a fork so they will break apart easily when baked. Bake at 350 degrees for 15-20 minutes.

CORN DODGERS
3 C corn meal
2 1/2 C boiling water
1 t salt

Mix ingredients and spoon onto floured cookie sheets. Form into desired shape. Bake at 375 degrees for about 30 minutes. Makes 10 Dodgers.

OAT DODGERS
3 C oats
1 C water
1 t salt, scant

Mix ingredients and shape into balls or ovals. Bake on floured cookie sheet at 300 degrees for 60 minutes. Yield: Approximately 20 balls.

DUMPLINGS
1/2 C water
1/2 t salt
2/3 C whole wheat flour

Place water and salt into a small pan and bring to a boil. Add flour. Stir until flour is absorbed and paste gathers into a ball. Cool until starch congeals and the dough "sets." Drop by teaspoonfuls into any stew or thick soup. Simmer 10 minutes.

FRENCH TOAST
1/4 C sesame seeds
2 1/2 C water
1/2 t salt
2 C oat flour
12 slices non-yeast bread (approx.)

Blend the first three ingredients in the blender. Pour this liquid into the flour and stir. Dip bread into the batter and bake at 400 degrees for 10 minutes. Reduce heat to 350 degrees until toast is nicely browned. Use broiler for last minute or two to brown the top.

WHOLE GRAINS

CORN FRITTERS
1 1/2 C whole kernel corn
1/4 C onions, chopped
1/3 C water
1/4 C wheat germ or bran
3/4 C plus 2 T whole grain flour or gluten flour
1/4 t salt

Lightly blend corn, onions and water in blender. Add other ingredients, mix, and drop by teaspoon onto floured cookie sheet. Bake at 350 degrees for 8-10 minutes or until golden brown on bottom, then bake for about 2 minutes in broiler until tops are golden brown.

HUSH PUPPIES
1 t salt
1 C grits (stoneground best)
1 C chopped onions
3-4 C water

Bring water to boil; add grits and salt. Cook for one hour. Cool until grits begin to get slightly stiff. It's important not to overcool. Add onions. Spoon onto floured baking sheet. Cool to congeal fully if not already stiff. Bake at 425 degrees for about 30-60 minutes. Give one minute under the broiler to get slightly browned if necessary.

SIMPLE CORN MUFFINS
1 1/2 C corn meal
1/4 C whole wheat flour
1 1/3 C water
1 t salt

Mix all ingredients. Let stand 20-30 minutes before shaping into muffins. Bake at 350 degrees for 45 min. Yield: 6 small muffins. May be baked in a pan and cut into squares for serving.

BASIC NOODLES
1 1/4 C whole wheat flour
1 C unbleached white flour
1 C warm water

Mix all ingredients well and roll out on a floured board to 1/8" thickness. Sprinkle with flour. Allow to dry for about half an hour (not necessary for lasagna noodles). Cut into 1 1/2" strips for lasagna noodles, 1/2" strips for macaroni or 1/4" strips for spaghetti. Noodles

WHOLE GRAINS

can be dried by hanging or laying at room temperature or by baking in a 200-degree oven until all trace of moisture is gone. Store in paper bag in cupboard.

POPOVERS

2 C whole grain flour
1 1/2 C water
1/4 C sesame seeds
1/2 t salt

Blend ingredients in blender until seeds are ground. Heat a floured muffin pan in oven at 425 degrees. Quickly spoon 2-3 tablespoons of batter in each muffin cup. Place in oven for 6-8 minutes. Then reduce heat to 375 degrees for about 8 minutes until the edges begin to brown. Toast 1-2 minutes under broiler to give a light brown color, watching carefully.

SPOON BREAD

2 C hot water
1 C sifted corn meal
1 t salt
2 C cooked or canned whole kernel corn

Blend and boil the above ingredients until thick. Add corn. Blend in blender until creamy. If mixture is too thick for the blender to handle, add a little water. Pour into flat, floured baking pan or casserole dish. Bake at 400 degrees for 1 1/2 hours or until golden brown. Keep the casserole dish covered until shortly before spoon bread is done. Serve hot or cold.

TORTILLAS

2 C fine corn meal
1 C water
1/2 t salt

Mix all ingredients into approximately six balls the size of a small apple. Roll each ball out, to desired thickness, between two sheets of waxed paper. Bake slowly in hot, ungreased, heavy iron skillet, turning to brown both sides. After cooling, these tortillas can be stacked and frozen.

(side tab) WHOLE GRAINS

Note: The dough will handle much easier if it is allowed to rest either before or after rolling into balls. Cover balls with an inverted bowl for 30-45 minutes, then roll out and bake.

MARIA'S TORTILLAS
2 C water
1 C oatmeal
1/4 C sesame seeds
4 C whole wheat flour
1/2 t salt

Blend water, oatmeal, and sesame seeds together in a blender until smooth. Pour into bowl, adding other ingredients. Knead. Place ball of dough under inverted bowl and let rest for 30-45 minutes. Roll out into small circles and bake on a hot griddle for 1 minute or so on each side.

POPCORN

Mostly considered a snack food, popcorn is actually very nourishing - 18% of its calories are protein. Popcorn can be served instead of bread at dinner, as a cereal for breakfast, or as a topping over cooked grain cereal. An air popper is ideal, however, the following method also works well:

1/3 C popcorn, dipped in salty water, then dried

Place a large, covered kettle or fry pan on the stove at moderately high heat. Put popcorn in the pan. Shake the pan gently so popcorn grains heat uniformly. Be prepared to pour into bowl as soon as popping ceases as the bottom kernels will burn.

Note: Unpopped kernels can be saved to grind in the blender and use in cooked cereals or roasts.

STEAMED WHOLE BARLEY
1 C whole barley, hulled
5 C water
1 t sea salt

Put all ingredients in the top of a double boiler, filling bottom with proper amount of water and using lid. Steam for 2 hours. Best prepared

227

at night and reheated in the morning. Leftover cold barley can be used for "Barley Burgers" below.

BARLEY BURGERS
2 C whole cooked barley
1/4 C grated raw potato
1/2 C finely ground seeds (optional)
2 t onion powder
1/4 t thyme
Salt to taste
Bread or waffle crumbs to form stiff burgers

Put barley through coarse food grinder or blend for a few seconds. Add all other ingredients, mixing well. Shape into flat burgers and brown both sides in a heavy skillet or in a broiler.

WHOLE BERRY CROCKPOT CEREAL
1 C berries (barley, wheat or rye)
1/2 C millet or rice
4 1/2 C water
1 1/4 t salt

Combine all ingredient in a crockpot and simmer overnight. (Some crockpots can accomplish this on a low or medium setting — other must be set on high. A high enough temperature to burst the shells of the grain must be achieved.)

DOSAS
1/2 C brown rice
1/2 C dried black beans
Salt to taste
Herbs to taste

Wash rice and beans, then soak overnight. Blend in blender with enough water to make a thin batter. Add salt and herbs, blending lightly. Let stand for a few minutes.

Place a griddle or frying pan over medium heat. Pour 1 tablespoon of batter on the griddle and quickly spread around to a crepe consistency. Turn over with a spatula and cook on the other side, making certain not to burn. Can be served with a sauce and steamed vegetables, or used to hold a filling like an enchilada.

WHOLE GRAINS

BUCKWHEAT RICE CEREAL
1/2 C buckwheat groats
5 C water
1 C brown rice
1 t salt

Combine all ingredients and boil for 1 1/2 hours. Due to the slightly strong flavor of buckwheat, it is best combined with a bland grain such as rice or millet.

BUCKWHEAT CRISPIES
1/2 C buckwheat groats
1/4 t salt
1 large onion, chopped
1 C boiling water
1 C (approx.) whole wheat or buckwheat flour
1 C water (approx.)

Dextrinize buckwheat groats for 5 minutes, stirring constantly. Add salt, onion, and boiling water. Cover and cook gently for 10 minutes. Remove from heat and add enough whole wheat or buckwheat flour and water to make either round balls from a stiff dough, or patties from a thinner dough. Bake on non-stick cookie sheet at 350 degrees for 20-25 minutes until crusty brown. Serve with vegetables.

HOMINY GRITS
1 C grits, stoneground
3-4 C water
1 t salt

Bring the water to a boil, then add grits and salt. Reduce heat and cook gently for 1-3 hours, the longer the better. (If, after 10 minutes of cooking, the grits look watery, add a few more grits so they do not turn out runny.) When finished cooking, they should be the consistency of mashed potatoes. Leftovers can be refrigerated, then sliced and baked for 1 hour at 350 degrees.

CORN MEAL MUSH
1 C cornmeal
3/4 C cold water
2 1/2 C boiling water
1/2 t salt

WHOLE GRAINS

Blend corn meal and cold water, then add to the boiling water, stirring until it boils. Let boil quite rapidly until it begins to thicken. Reduce the heat to low and simmer for 20-40 minutes. Extra cooked mush can be stored in the refrigerator in molds and baked in slices.

CORN MEAL SOUFFLÉ

2 C boiling water
1/3 C corn meal
1/4 C gluten flour
3/4 t salt
1/4 C water

Pour boiling water over the corn meal. Cook in the double boiler for 30 minutes, stirring occasionally. Mix the water, salt and gluten flour and mix with the hot corn meal. Bake in baking dish about 1 hour at 350 degrees.

COOKED MILLET

1 C whole millet
4 C water
1 t salt

Combine ingredients and cook slowly two hours. Leftover cooked millet can be placed in storage containers in the refrigerator until cold and congealed. Slice in 1/3"- 1/2" slices and bake at 350 degrees for 45-60 minutes or toast.

OAT BURGERS OR LOAF

1 raw potato
1/2 C onion
Water
2 C cooked oatmeal
1-2 C bread or waffle crumbs
1 t salt
1/2 t sage

Blend cut up potato, onion and a little water in blender. Remove from blender and add remaining ingredients and mix. Add more crumbs, if necessary, to form patties or make into a roast. Bake in tin at 350 degrees until nicely browned. Burgers require 45 minutes, turning after 30 minutes. Loaf requires about 60 minutes.

WHOLE GRAINS

BAKED RICE
2 1/2 C brown rice
3 3/4 - 4 C water
1/2 t salt

Dextrinize rice in a deep fry pan on top of the stove until a golden brown. Place in a covered casserole with water and salt. Bake for 45 minutes in a 350-degree oven. Remove from oven and allow to cool a bit before serving.

RICE BALLS
Quantity of cooked rice, stirred vigorously to make creamy

Dip hands in salted water, then mold creamy rice into balls. Place on non-stick floured baking sheet and bake for 10 minutes at 450 degrees. A small piece of vegetable may be enclosed in the center of each ball.

FLAKY RICE
1 C rice
2 1/2 C water, heated
1/2 t salt

Toast rice in a dry pan on burner while stirring constantly, or in oven at 350 degrees for 15 to 20 minutes, until it turns golden brown and begins to pop. Pour immediately into preheated water. Be careful since the water will boil vigorously as the toasted rice is poured in. Reduce heat and barely simmer for 1-2 hours. Do not stir during any of the cooking period even though some may stick to the bottom.

When finished cooking, and all kernels are soft and well cooked, turn out carefully onto a platter to prevent its becoming creamy. To remove the crust which may sometimes stick to the bottom, simply add a small amount of water and cover the pot for a few minutes. Then lift the crust out with a spatula. Cut the crust in wedges and serve as wafers.

Note: It is better to cook Flaky Rice in a large flat pan such as an electric fry pan rather than a small diameter, deep kettle as the deeper layers tend to get more creamy as the depth of the rice increases.

WHOLE GRAINS

DRY RICE
1 C brown rice
3 C water
1 1/2 t salt

Preheat water, adding rice and salt. Cook very slowly for 1 1/4 hours without stirring. Turn out into a serving bowl by loosening with a spatula and dumping to avoid crushing the rice. This makes a fluffier, less creamy rice due to less stirring.

SPANISH RICE
1/2 C onion, chopped
1/2 C green pepper, chopped
1/2 t onion salt
2 C water
3/4 C tomato paste or cooked tomatoes
3 C cooked dry rice
1 C cooked garbanzo (chickpea) beans

Combine all but last two ingredients. Simmer gently until thickened, about 3-5 minutes. Add rice and garbanzos. Bake in floured casserole 25 minutes at 350 degrees.

RISOTTO MILANESE
1 1/2 C brown rice
6 C water or vegetable broth
1 t basil
1/2 C chopped onion
2 crushed buds garlic
1 1/2 t salt
1/2 t saffron, steeped in 3 T hot water, or 1 t paprika

Dextrinize the rice in a dry skillet on low heat for approx. 8 minutes, stirring continuously. Add the broth very carefully, then the basil, onion, garlic, and salt. Add drained saffron after steeping for 15 minutes, or use paprika. Cook rice slowly for about 1-2 hours, adding more broth if necessary.

WHOLE GRAINS

RICE AND LENTIL LOAF
2 C dry rice
1 C lentil pureé*
1 T onion
3 T water
2 T whole grain flour, browned
Sprinkle of sage
Salt to taste

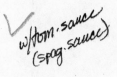

w/tom. sauce
(spag. sauce)

Mix all ingredients and pack lightly in a floured bread tin. Bake at 350 degrees for about 45 minutes or until slightly brown on top.

* Lentil pureé is made by combining 4 cups of cooked lentils and approximately 1/2 cup of water, then blend well.

WAFFLES

Waffles have long been known as a breakfast food, usually topped with a sweet topping and heavy butter or cream. However, waffles can also be healthy if one substitutes whole grain flour for white flour and eliminates high-sugar and fat toppings. Easy to prepare, freeze and reheat, waffles are probably the most versatile of all bread replacements. Use them for sandwiches, dried into crackers for dips and spreads, or in place of toast. Waffles can also be baked, cooled, stacked, and frozen. They reheat quickly in a toaster or at room temperature. If serving several people, put waffles on the rack of a 175-degree oven to keep warm. They can also be baked in an oven at 200 degrees until "dried" to a cracker consistency. Excellent for traveling.

It may take a little time and practice to master waffle making, but the results are worth it. Use a good *Silverstone* or non-stick waffle iron, preferably one with a temperature control (See Chapter 6, Tools For Kitchen Organization.) Set waffle iron on medium high and let pre-heat. Follow the easy directions below:

1. Using proportions of any of the following recipes, put liquid ingredients into blender first, then flour. Do not overfill. Blend ingredients *thoroughly*, adding more water or flour as needed to achieve a nice "pancake" type batter. Abundant blending is the secret to "light" waffles! If the batter thickens between batches, simply add a little more water and reblend. Always use *hot water and/or hot cooked grain to make waffle batter.*

2. When waffle iron is hot, pour batter into each waffle section, being careful not to overfill. Let batter set a minute before slowly lowering the lid of the waffle iron.

3. Bake 10-15 minutes (without raising lid) or until steam no longer escapes from the sides of the waffle iron.

GARBANZO WAFFLES

1 C cooked garbanzos
1 1/2 C rolled oats
2-4 t seeds (optional)
1/2 t salt
2 1/4 C hot water

Blend all ingredients thoroughly in blender. Bake as directed.

OAT WAFFLES

8 C rolled oats, lightly dextrinized in oven
1 T salt
8 C hot water

Mix together and allow to stand overnight in refrigerator. Bake as directed.

POPCORN WAFFLES

2 C unbolted corn flour
2 C water
2 1/4 C popped popcorn
1/2 - 1 t salt
1 1/4 C hot water

Blend corn flour and 2 cups water in blender and let set for at least one hour. Blend 2 minutes more, adding remaining ingredients. *blend well*. Let set 10 minutes. Reblend slightly and pour into hot iron. If the batter is too thick to pour nicely over the grids, add up to 1/4 cup more water and blend again.

QUANTITY RICE WAFFLES

1 1/3 C brown rice flour
3/4 C water
1 C hot water
1/2 C cooked brown rice
1/4 C seeds (optional)
1/2 - 1 t salt

Combine brown rice flour and 3/4 cup water, stirring to make a paste. Let sit for at least one hour. Put paste in the blender with rest of ingredients. Blend thoroughly. Additional water may be necessary. Pour gently into waffle iron and bake as directed.

RICE AND SEED WAFFLES
1 C uncooked long-grain brown rice
1 1/2 C water
1/4 - 1/2 C sesame seeds (optional)
1/2 C cooked brown rice
1 1/4 C hot water
1/2 - 1 t salt

Soak overnight (or at least two hours), 1 cup long grain brown rice and 1 1/2 cups water. Thoroughly blend with 1/4-1/2 cup sesame seeds (three minutes or more). Add cooked brown rice, 1 1/4 cups water, and salt. Blend again. Pour gently into waffle iron and bake as directed.

WHOLE GRAINS

VEGETABLES

GREEN LIMA BEANS WITH FINE HERBS
2 pkgs (10 oz each) frozen green limas
1 t lemon juice
1 T chopped chives
1 T minced parsley
1 t tarragon
Salt to taste

Cook lima beans in small amount of water until tender (30 to 45 minutes). Add rest of ingredients and serve as a main dish.

CORN STEW
1 - 1 1/2 C whole corn
3 onions, chopped
3 green peppers, chopped
3 tomatoes, quartered
Salt to taste

Simmer onions, tomatoes and peppers gently for 5 minutes. Add corn and simmer for 5-10 minutes. Salt to taste.

STUFFED PEPPERS
5 medium bell peppers
4 C Spanish Rice (recipe in Grain section)

Cut peppers in half, remove seeds and stems. Cook by steaming in a little water in a large kettle for about ten minutes. Stuff each half with the rice mixture. Place in a floured, covered baking dish at 350 degrees for 30 minutes. Uncover and brown for 1 minute under the broiler.

NOTE: Green peppers can also be stuffed with any mixture, such as beans-rice-tomato sauce-olives, or a vegetable medley with hummus.

COUNTRY POTATO PATTIES
6 med. potatoes, boiled or baked
2 T minced onion
2 T chopped pimento or celery
1 T chopped parsley
2 T flour (whole wheat, oat, etc.)
Salt to taste

VEGATABLES

Shred potatoes with coarse grater. Mix with all other ingredients. Shape into patties or mounds. Brown in oven on *Silverstone* cookie sheet.

FRENCH FRIES

Slice raw potatoes into french fry shapes leaving skins on. Place on *Silverstone* cookie sheet. Bake for 40 minutes at 375 degrees, or until done. Watch closely. Should be slightly brown on the outside and tender inside.

VICKI'S MASHED POTATOES
Cooked potatoes, with skins
Grain milk (recipe in Miscellaneous section)
Salt to taste

Make certain potatoes are well-cooked. Use approx. 1-1 1/2 potatoes for each serving. Mash potatoes, mixing in enough grain milk to achieve desired consistency. Salt to taste.

SHEPHERD PIE
2 C diced onions sauteed in water
2 C diced, cooked carrots
2 C potatoes, cooked with skins
2 C cooked beans — *any*
Mashed potatoes for icing

Place all vegetables and 1 cup of the beans in a deep casserole dish. Puree the second cup of beans, adding enough water to thin down. Pour pureed bean mixture over vegetables, filling about 1/3 of the dish. Spread mashed potatoes on top as an icing. Heat in the oven for about 30 minutes before serving. Lightly brown the icing peaks. Serve as a single dish with green onions and carrot strips.

HOT POTATO SALAD
2 T minced onion
1 t parsley flakes
1 C mock sour cream (recipe in Miscellaneous section)
1 t salt
4 C hot cooked potato cubes

Combine all ingredients except hot potato cubes. Heat, if desired, but do not boil. Pour over hot potatoes and toss.

VEGETABLES

SQUASH TAMALE BAKE

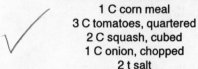

1 C corn meal
3 C tomatoes, quartered
2 C squash, cubed
1 C onion, chopped
2 t salt

Place the ingredients together in a saucepan, stirring until squash has released its juice well, and corn meal has thickened. Cook on stovetop for approximately 15 minutes. Put in baking dish and continue baking in oven at 350 degrees for about 1 hour.

ZUCCHINI AND ONIONS
Equal amounts of zucchini and onions

Shred zucchini squash finely, using a grater. Add equal quantities of chopped onions. Place in a deep kettle on medium heat. (Makes its own liquid for steaming.) Steam until tender. Serve with small amount of salt.

VEGATABLES

MISCELLANEOUS RECIPES

DIGESTIVE DRINKS

CABBAGE JUICE

Cabbage juice should be used twice per day, immediately before the first and second meal (do not use with a third meal). Approximately 1/2 hour before these meals, set a head of cabbage out to warm slightly at room temperature. Then, immediately before eating, cut cabbage and put enough through a juicer to make approximately four ounces (a glass measuring cup under the spigot works nicely). Shut juicer off and let finish filling for a couple seconds. No more than 4-6 ounces of cabbage juice is needed. 3-C Helpers may be added at this time. *Drink immediately out of the juicer as the healing benefits of cabbage juice oxidize very rapidly.* Follow immediately with meal.

PARSLEY-PINEAPPLE DRINK

Pour only four ounces of pineapple juice (frozen is preferred over canned if fresh is not available) into a measuring cup and add approximately one-half cup of fresh, washed parsley. Put in blender and turn blender on *only long enough* to "break" the parsley (one or two seconds). Drink immediately upon preparation, adding any 3-C Helpers. Follow immediately with meal.

MILK REPLACEMENTS

GRAIN MILK

Any cooked grain can be used in making grain milk. Simply fill a blender with hot water. Add one cup of hot, cooked grain. Blend until the grain has been thoroughly liquified (this may take several minutes). Pour through fine strainer to remove any remaining small particles. Adjust amounts of grain and water to suit individual taste.

Grain milk is an excellent replacement for those allergic to cow's milk. It is also easier to digest than soy or nut milk. In the 3-C Program, it can be used in recipes such as mashed potatoes.

MISCELLANEOUS

Rice milk can be made following the directions in "Grain Milk," or try this variation:

RICE MILK
2 C water
1 C rice flour

Combine water and flour and blend in blender. Cook for 1-3 hours in a double boiler. Store in refrigerator. To make milk, place one cup of rice base in blender. Add sufficient water to make the consistency of milk. Can be thickened by adding more rice base or cooked whole grains. Blend very well.

CHEESE REPLACEMENTS

AGAR CHEESE - (A cheese that will melt)
1/4 - 1/2 C agar (see this section)
1 1/2 C water
3/4 C sesame seeds
1/4 - 1/2 C pimentos
1 t salt
1 t onion or garlic
2-4 T lemon juice

Soak agar in water about 5 minutes and boil gently until clear. While agar is boiling, place the next five ingredients in blender and blend until smooth. Add hot agar and blend 30 seconds. Add the lemon juice last and mix only for a second. Pour immediately into molds and set in refrigerator to cool. Slice thinly or cut into cubes.

PASTA CHEESE SAUCE - (Excellent for blending)
1 C tomatoes or 1/2 C pimentos
1 C water
1/3 C lemon juice (or as desired)
1 1/2 t salt
1/8 t garlic powder

Blend all ingredients in a blender until smooth. Heat just until hot, then serve.

CHEESE TOPPER - (Ideal for pouring over vegetables)
1/2 C potatoes, well cooked
3/4 C hot water
1/4 C pimentos
1-3 T lemon juice
1/2 t salt

Blend all ingredients until smooth, then heat. May substitute 1 cup tomatoes for pimentos and water. Excellent over vegetables, grain dishes, loaves, etc.

BUTTER REPLACEMENTS

FRESH CORN BUTTER
1 C fresh or frozen corn, cooked
1/3 t salt
2 T water

Blend all ingredients until smooth. Use as butter.

MILLET OR RICE BUTTER
1 C hot rice or millet
1/2 - 1 1/2 C water
1/2 - 1 t salt (or more to taste)

Blend all ingredients well. May add garlic or onion or lemon juice. Dilute to use as a cream or salad dressing.

DRESSINGS/TOPPINGS

MOCK "SOUR CREAM"
1 1/3 C sunflower seeds
1 2/3 C water
1 t salt
1/3 C lemon juice (or as desired)
1/4 t garlic powder
1/2 t onion powder

Blend all ingredients to a smooth consistency. Can be used as a topping for potatoes or thinned down with water for a salad dressing. Keep in mind that the sunflower seeds are concentrated, so use sparingly. For instance, thin down and pour over potatoes as a main dish. May have to have a little more water added and reblend if left standing.

MISCELLANEOUS

FRENCH DRESSING
1/4 C lemon juice
1 C fresh or canned tomatoes
2 t paprika
1 t salt

Thoroughly blend all ingredients in a blender. May be further seasoned with mild herbs. Store in a glass jar in refrigerator.

SUNNY TOMATO DRESSING
1 C fresh or canned tomatoes
1/2-1 C sunflower seeds
1 t garlic powder
2 t onion power
1/4 C lemon juice
1/2 t salt

Thoroughly blend all ingredients. Will thicken upon standing. Seed quantity may be reduced. Eat sparingly of this dressing due to the seed content. Store in glass jar in refrigerator.

DRESSINGS
1 fresh vegetable
1 T lemon juice
1/2 t salt
Water as needed

Any vegetable (depending on preference) can be blended with lemon juice and salt until smooth. If onions, peppers, cucumbers, radishes, or certain other vegetables are used, water may be added in the blender to achieve desired consistency. Serve over any vegetable salad.

GRAVIES

Due to the various items in gravies, remember to limit the number of items at each meal. If, for example, seasoned or brown gravy was being served, the main dish could consist of rice and potatoes, since those gravies do not contain too many items. However, the tomato gravy has a few more, so serving it over rice only would be better; simply eat several servings.

SEASONED GRAVY
2 C water
1 t onion powder
1/4 C browned flour (whole wheat, barley, rice)
1/4 t any mixed herbs
1/2 t salt

Blend all ingredients in blender. Place in saucepan and cook until done (about 10 minutes). Serve with vegetarian roasts or burgers and as stock for many stews, casseroles, and baked vegetables.

BROWN GRAVY
1/2 C whole grain flour
Salt to taste
2 C vegetable broth or water

Dextrinize flour until entirely browned. Cool slightly by rubbing the outside of the pan with a wet cloth. Add one-third of the liquid, and stir until smooth, with no lumps. Add the rest of the liquid and let boil slowly for 10 minutes. For variation, sauté chopped onions in a little water first, then add to liquid. If smooth texture is desired, return to the blender and blend until creamy.

TOMATO GRAVY
2 C tomatoes
1 sm. onion
1/2 clove garlic
2 stalks celery, chopped fine
1 t salt
1/4 C whole grain flour
1/4 C cold water

Simmer the first four items for 5 minutes. Make a paste using the flour and water. Add to the tomatoes. Simmer slowly over very low heat for 10-20 minutes. One half bay leaf may be added if desired. If a smooth gravy is preferred, blend just before serving.

BEAN GRAVY
Leftover beans, peas, split peas, lentils, garbanzos
Water or grain milk
Desired seasonings

MISCELLANEOUS

Place 1-2 cups beans in blender with enough water and/or grain milk to make the desired consistency. Season with onion, garlic, salt, herbs, etc.

RICE GRAVY
1-2 C hot rice
1-2 C water
1/4 C sunflower seeds, toasted

Toast seeds in dry skillet on stovetop. Place toasted seeds, rice and water in blender and blend until smooth, adding more water if a thinner consistency is desired. Can be poured over cooked rice at breakfast, over biscuits, etc.

SPREADS/DIPS

HUMMUS
3 C cooked garbanzos (chickpeas)
1/2 C Tahini or 3/4 C sesame seeds
1 clove garlic (optional)
5 T lemon juice
1 t salt
Water

Pureé all ingredients with enough water to achieve a smooth consistency. Excellent on any bread-type item. Can also be thinned down for a gravy or salad dressing. (There are many different versions of this delicious Eastern staple, each one varying by one or two ingredients. Experiment with amounts and ingredients until favorite proportions are achieved.)

GUACAMOLE
1 avocado
1/2 medium tomato, diced
1 T lemon juice
1/2 t garlic salt

Mash avocado and add to other ingredients. Blend thoroughly. Chill and serve. Avocados are concentrated, so use this recipe sparingly.

SEASONINGS

NON-IRRITATING CURRY POWDER
1 t paprika
1 T ground coriander
1 T dill seed
1 T garlic powder

Mix. Store tightly closed. Use in any recipe calling for curry.

GOMASIO SEASONING
1 C unhulled sesame seeds 1/2 t salt

As explained in Chapter 5, herbs are the leafy parts of plants that do not typically cause irritation, as can spices. However, some herbs are very strong. The herbs listed below are mild herbs which are safe to use as seasonings in limited quantities.

Herbs gradually lose flavor and color during storage. They should not be purchased in large quantities and should be stored in airtight containers in a cool, dry place out of direct light.

MILD HERBS PERMITTED ON 3-C PROGRAM

Basil	Fennel Seed	Onion	Saffron
Bay Leaf	Garlic	Paprika	Sage
Coriander	Marjoram	Parsley	Sesame Seed
Dill Seed	Mint	Rosemary	Tarragon
Thyme	Caraway Seed	Chives	Savory

Gently roast sesame seeds in a dry skillet until they are *lightly* browned. Add salt and grind *briefly*, using a seed grinder or a blender. Excellent on salads, rice, vegetables, entrees and burgers.

AGAR, AGAR

Agar, agar is a tasteless, seaweed (algae) which is non-irritating, absorbs moisture rapidly, and retains it. It is used as a jelling agent in salads, soups and desserts, in place of animal gelatin. It jells readily at room temperature and a little goes a long way. Approximate basic

MISCELLANEOUS

proportions: 3 1/2 cups liquid to 2 T flakes or 3 1/2 cups liquid to 1 T granules.

ARROWROOT POWDER

Arrowroot powder is a pure, nutritious starch made from the beaten pulp of the tuberous rootstocks of an American tropical plant. It yields an easily digestible starch with a calcium ash and some trace minerals. Arrowroot can be used in place of cornstarch to thicken fruits, soups, gravies, etc. Basic proportions: 1 cup liquid to 1 1/2 tablespoon arrowroot powder. Dissolve arrowroot in a little *cold* water first, then add to liquid. Bring to a boil to thicken.

RICE FLOUR OR POWDER

Dextrinize brown rice by roasting in a dry skillet, stirring constantly until golden and it begins to pop, or place in a 350 degree oven for 15-20 minutes. Blend at high speed in blender until it becomes a powder, or grind in a mill. Use for thickening stews and gravies, as a binder in casseroles, or for cream of rice.

HYDROGEN PEROXIDE (H_2O_2)

Hydrogen peroxide (food-grade quality only) can be used in place of baking soda, baking powder or yeast for rising purposes. The extra ion of oxygen in hydrogen peroxide is liberated, causing the baked item to rise somewhat. Hydrogen peroxide can be used in most any recipe such as cake, cookies, waffles, etc. After baking thoroughly, no hydrogen peroxide taste will remain as it dissipates totally during the baking process.

Food-grade quality hydrogen peroxide should be used for cooking since the drug-store variety may contain undesirable chemicals. However, whereas drug-store hydrogen peroxide is a 3 percent solution, food-grade hydrogen peroxide is a 35 percent concentrate. Before cooking with food-grade hydrogen peroxide, first find out whether the recipe amounts call for a 3 percent or a 35 percent solution. For example, if a recipe calls for 1/4 to 1/3 cup of H_2O_2, they are referring to the weaker 3 percent solution. To convert the 35 percent into the customary 3 percent solution, *Mix one part 35 percent food-grade hydrogen peroxide with 11 parts distilled water.* It may take some experimenting to determine exactly how much food-grade hydrogen peroxide is required for certain recipes.

Hydrogen peroxide can also be used as an effective wash for vegetables and fruits. Use 1/4 cup of 3 percent hydrogen peroxide to a sink of tepid water. Soak thick skinned items 20-30 minutes, then rinse and drain. Lighter items like leafy greens and lettuce can be soaked for 15-20 minutes. Hydrogen peroxide does not produce fumes so common with *Clorox* food baths.

A WORD ABOUT SOUPS

Soups are easy, convenient, and economical to fix. However, there are a few guidelines when using soups in the 3-C Program:

1) Limit number of items in soup to four. This does not include garlic, onions, or a couple of seasonings.

2) Use the least amount of liquid needed to prepare soup. Rather than a soup, a "stew" consistency is desired. If a cooked soup has too much liquid, simply drain some off, reserving it for vegetable stock.

3) To thicken soups, remove one cup of the cooked vegetables and one cup of the liquid. Put both in blender and pureé, adding back into the soup to thicken. Also, cooked potatoes can be pureéd and added to soup to thicken.

4) Soups are a great place to "hide" a least-liked vegetable or bean, especially when serving children. The item can be cooked, then pureed in a blender with a little of the soup stock. Add to soup. This is especially ideal with broccoli, spinach, cabbage, brussel sprouts, etc.

5) When first learning to cook a new way, some failures are bound to occur. A soup is an excellent place to blend in a "flopped" recipe that is otherwise perfectly safe to eat. Keep in mind to limit amount of ingredients. For instance, if a recipe for "Country Potato Patties" did not work out the first time, it could be blended into a pot of potato soup. Use more of the same herbs and seasonings (onion, parsley, celery, salt), which will limit the number of items.

MISCELLANEOUS

Purchasing and Storing Pineapple

Ripe pineapple should have a golden or golden-orange skin color. When tapping it, a hollow sound indicates that it is not yet ripe. Instead, it should feel heavy and solid when thumped. After cutting, fresh pineapple does not keep very long, usually a few days in the refrigerator. Store in a covered container.

Purchasing And Storing Avocados

It often takes a little time and patience to cultivate a knack for choosing good avocados, but the taste is worth it. A good avocado should be heavy for its size, with no indentations, open cracks or dark bruises. Avocados that are ripe will have a darker skin and should be soft enough to "give" when pressed with the thumb. If not, they can easily be ripened at room temperature in a few days or even more quickly if placed in a paper bag. Store at room temperature until ripe, then refrigerate. Once the flesh is exposed to air, it will quickly darken unless lemon juice is added.

To properly peel an avocado, wash and cut in two, twisting apart. Remove pit. The avocado can now be peeled and sliced to put on sandwiches, as a beautiful garnish, or side vegetable. Or, the flesh can be spooned out and mashed to use in a variety of recipes such as guacamole. Serve with vegetables, crackers, or corn chips (there are no-oil varieties available in health food stores or they can be home-baked). Avocado can also take the place of butter, making an excellent spread on rice cakes, crackers, and waffles.

MISCELLANEOUS

RECEIPE SOURCES

Many of the recipes in this book were adapted from those contained in the books below:

A GOOD COOK...TEN TALENTS

BROWN RICE COOKBOOK

COUNTRY LIFE NATURAL FOODS

NUTRITION SEMINAR COOKBOOK

EAT FOR STRENGTH COOKBOOK OIL FREE EDITION

OF THESE YE MAY FREELY EAT

RECIPES FROM THE WEIMAR KITCHEN

WHOLE FOODS FOR WHOLE PEOPLE

REFERENCES AND RECOMMENDED READING

It is my personal belief that every adult should intelligently take charge of their own health. We need to factilitate this by reading, studying, and learning before we make decisions. The books listed below can provide much more additional information either as a reference point or in substantiating foundations of the 3-C Program.

Yeast Connection, 3rd Edition, Dr. William Crook, Professional Books, Jackson, TN, 1987.

The Missing Diagnosis, Dr. C.O. Truss, Birmingham, Alabama.

Candida: A Twentieth Century Disease, Shirley Lorenzani, Ph.D., Keats Publishing, New Canaan, CT , 1986.

Yeast Syndrome, Dr. John Trowbridge, Bantam Books, New York, NY, 1986. Vicki's abbreviated story appears in this book on page 55 under the name Sally Whiteburn.

Nutrition For Vegetarians, Drs Calvin and Agatha Thrash, Newlifestyle Books, Seale, AL, 1982.

Food Facts, A Compendium On Whole Foods, Evelyn Roehl, Food Learning Center, Seattle, WA 1986.

Nutrition Almanac, Nutrition Search, Inc., McGraw-Hill Books, New York, N.Y., 1975

Composition Of Foods, United States Department of Agriculture, Washington, D.C., 1984

Super Calorie, Carbohydrate Counter, Richard Passwater, Ph.D., Dale Books, NY, 1978.

The Animal Connection, Drs. Agatha and Calvin Thrash, Newlifestyle Books, Seale, AL, 1983.

Unsafe At Any Meal, Earl Mindell, Warner Books, New York, N.Y., 1987.

Modern Meat, Antibiotics, Hormones & The Pharmaceutical Farm, Orville Schell, Random, 1985.

Diet For A New America: How Your Food Choices Affect Your Health, Happiness And The Future Of Life On Earth, John Robbins, Stillpoint, 1987.

Home Remedies, Drs. Calvin and Agatha Thrash, Newlifestyle Books, Seale, AL, 1981

Hydrotherapy, Dr. Dail and Thomas, TEACH Services, Brushton, NY, 1989.

Rx, Charcoal, Drs. Calvin and Agatha Thrash, Newlifestyle Books, Seale, AL, 1988

Sunlight, Zane R. Kime, M.D., M.S., World Health Publications, Penryn, CA, 1980.

The Choice Is Clear, Allen E. Banik, M.D., Acres USA, 1975.

Report On Water, H.W. Holderby, M.D. Natural Food Associates, Atlanta, Texas, 75551

Healthy Water For A Longer Life, Martin Fox, Ph.D., *Troubled Water*, Jonathan King and *Elixir Of The Ageless*, Patrick Flanagan and Gael Crystal Flanagan, Acres USA, Kansas City, Missouri.

The Shocking Truth About Water, Paul C. Bragg and Patricia Bragg, Health Science, 25th edition.

The 20th Century Principle, David A. Elliott, Green World Publications, Ferndale, WA.

Health Freedom Newsletter, "Flouradation, Good or Bad?", May, 1987.

Human Circadian Rhythms, J.N. Mills, Physiological Review, Vol 146, No 1, 1966.

Biologic Rhythms And Hormone Secretion Patterns, E.D. Weitzman, Hospital Practice, Aug 1976.

Some Aspects Of Circadian Variations Of Carbohydrate Metabolism And Related Hormones In Man, S. Sensi, Chronobiologia, Vol 1, No 4 Oct-Dec 1974.

Biological Rhythms And Human Performance, W. P. Colquhoun, Academic Press, 1971.

The Body Clock Diet, R. Gatty, Ph.D., Simon and Schuster. 1978.

Emphasis Your Health, Dr. Thrash, Vol. 7-3., 1991.

A Randomized Double-blind Trial Of Nystatin Therapy For The Candidiasis Hypersensitivity Syndrome, William E. Dismukes, J. Scott Wade, Jeannette Y. Lee, Bonita K. Dockery, and Jack D. Hain. *New England Journal Of Medicine #25,* 12/90, Vol. 323, pg 1717.

The New York Times, "eating To Heal; The New Frontiers", Feb. 7, 1990.

The Mcdougall Plan, John A. McDougall, M.D. & Mary McDougall, New Centrury Publishers, Inc., 1983

Nutrient Information was taken from food composition tables from the United States Department of Agriculture's *"Composition of Foods",* most recently revised edition. Not all nutrient values were available for all foods. Also, nutritional analyses represent data for certain tested foods and nutritional contents vary due to soil, weather, processing, storage conditions and individual metabolism.

Iron chart taken from Drause and Hunscher, *Food, Nutrition and Diet Therapy,*W.B. Saunders, 1972, adapted in *"Nutrition for Vegetarians."*

Calcium chart adapted from *"Vibrant Life,"* 3/89.

Chart showing lose of nutrients of whole wheat take from *"Lesser Known Vitamins in Foods,"* Journal of American Dietary Assoc., 38, 1961.

*"Beloved, I wish above all things
that thou mayest prosper
and be in health."* 3 John 2